DIABETES
Survival
Guide

DIABETES
Survival
Guide

UNDERSTANDING THE FACTS ABOUT DIAGNOSIS, TREATMENT, AND PREVENTION

Originally published as
CONTROLLING DIABETES THE EASY WAY

STANLEY MIRSKY, M.D., AND JOAN RATTNER HEILMAN

BALLANTINE BOOKS · NEW YORK

This book cannot and must not replace hands-on medical care or the specific advice of your doctor. Use it instead to help you ask the right questions, make the right choices, and work more closely with your doctor and other members of your health-care team.

To Susan, Jennifer, and Jonathan

Also to the memory of my mentor,
Dr. Elliot P. Joslin, 1869–1962.
Gladly would he learn, and gladly teach.

And to the memory of my twin brother,
who lived for fifty-five years with
diabetes without complications.

CONTENTS

1

WHAT IT MEANS TO BE A DIABETIC

Nobody is delighted to be diagnosed as a diabetic. After all, diabetes is a chronic disease with serious consequences and complications if it isn't kept under control. You must watch what you eat, get regular exercise, and maybe take pills or insulin injections. It is a condition that you will have for the rest of your days. So far, there is no cure.

But diabetes is the one major disorder whose effects on your lifestyle depend to a remarkable degree on how much you know, and how much effort and time you are willing to spend paying attention to it. You can minimize the impact it has on your daily life as well as your future health simply by learning all about it and then living with a few rules that actually would make everyone in the world healthier if they, too, abided by them. At best, you may lose all evidence of diabetes and indeed the disease itself. At least, you may be able to reduce the amount of medication you require—all as the result of eating sensibly. The easy-to-follow plan presented here may change your life.

About 21 million Americans, 7 percent of the population, have diabetes, although many of them are not aware of it. Another 47 million, including 2 million adolescents ages twelve to nineteen, have prediabetes, a condition that may lead to type 2 diabetes later in life. The prevalence of the disease nearly doubled in the American adult population from 1990 to 2002 and has risen by more than 14 percent since 2003. In adults older than sixty, nearly one in every five has diabetes, and the incidence is rapidly rising in children and adolescents.

Studies estimate the cost of diabetes to be over $132 billion a year, some in direct costs, including hospitalization and treatment, and the rest in lost productivity, disability payments, loss of work time, and premature deaths. Diabetes consumes $1 out of every $10 spent on health care in the United States.

To give you all the bad news at once, Diabetes is the only major disease with a death rate that is still rising. Diabetics are much more likely than others to become blind, lose a foot or a leg, have kidney failure, develop coronary heart disease and stroke. In addition, it is now thought that they are twice as likely to develop Alzheimer's disease.

Now for the good news. Tremendous progress has been made in only the last few years in the prevention and treatment of the disease. It is very likely that a cure will be discovered soon. Most diabetics who not long ago would have died at an early age or would have existed with such dire complications that life would have been hardly worth living, can now lead almost normal lives and can look forward to a respectable, reasonably healthy old age.

THE FACTS ABOUT DIABETES

• More than nine out of ten of the diagnosed diabetics in the United States have type 2, or noninsulin-dependent diabetes mellitus (NIDDM). If they follow the correct diet, this group—formerly known as "adult-onset diabetics" because the disease usually strikes adults over the age of forty and most commonly over fifty-five—may never need insulin injections except perhaps during periods of stress. The remaining less than 10 percent of diagnosed diabetics have type 1, or insulin-dependent diabetes mellitus (IDDM). Once called "juvenile-onset diabetics" because it typically strikes in childhood, this group will always require insulin and cannot get along with diet alone or even with oral antidiabetic agents. Type 1 and type 2 are two separate disorders, although they share many of the very same problems.

• In the U.S. each year, over thirteen thousand children are diagnosed with type 1 diabetes. And more and more children and teens have type 2, with some clinics reporting that one-third to one-half of all new cases of childhood diabetes are now type 2. According to the American Heart Association, those at especially high risk are African American, Latino, Asian American, and Native American Indian children who are obese and have a family history of type 2.

• All type 1 diabetics require insulin injections because they make little or no insulin themselves.

• Ten to 20 percent of the diagnosed type 2 diabetics are treated with diet and exercise. Thirty to 40 percent take oral drugs to keep their blood sugar within acceptable limits. And 30 to 40 percent require insulin injections or a combination of insulin and oral medications.

• Type 1 diabetes is more prevalent among whites than other racial groups.

• About 11 percent of white Americans ages forty-five to seventy-four have type 2 diabetes, according to the National Institutes of Health. Among African Americans, however, the rate is over 18 percent in the same age range and black women are particularly vulnerable;

one in four over the age of fifty-five has diabetes. The forecast is even bleaker for Latinos, especially Mexican Americans and Puerto Ricans, who suffer from diabetes at twice the rate of whites. There is a disproportionately high prevalence of the disease, more than twice that of U.S. adults overall, in Native American and Alaska Native adults. This is true, too, of Asian Americans who have abandoned their traditional foods and adopted a Western diet, high in fat and sugar. They are particularly susceptible to type 2 diabetes and often develop it at much lower weights than people of other races.

• The chances of developing diabetes double with every 20 percent of excess weight and with every ten years of increasing age. They also increase with the accumulation of fat around the middle. A recent study suggests that men with a waist size of 40 inches or more have the highest risk of type 2 diabetes, twelve times more likely than those with a size of 34 inches or less.

• Two in three people with diabetes will develop heart disease. Nearly 80 percent of diabetics die of heart disease or stroke. Adult diabetics are two to four times more likely to have a heart attack or stroke than other people, the same risk as if they have already had a heart attack, according to the American Diabetes Association.

• Gender matters. Before menopause, women have built-in protection against heart attacks, but they lose that protection if they have diabetes.

THE DIABETES EPIDEMIC

Diabetes in the United States has reached epidemic proportions, with over a million new cases diagnosed every year. What's more, although type 2 diabetes mostly continues to strike older people, more children and teenagers are getting it and much of the blame has been attributed to the long hours they spend in front of the computer or the TV set instead of on their feet.

America's children are growing fatter. The Centers for Disease Control estimates that one in three Americans born in the year 2000 will develop diabetes in their lifetime. Women and minorities face the greatest risk.

WHAT IS DIABETES?

Diabetes mellitus is a metabolic disorder that results in persistent *hyper*glycemia—an abnormally high amount of sugar in the blood. (On the other hand, *hypoglycemia* means the opposite—an abnormally *low* blood-sugar level.) It is thought today that diabetes is actually several different diseases with different causes, all with the same result: the inability of the body to efficiently utilize the carbohydrates we eat as a source of fuel.

Glucose, the sugar molecule that is the end product of carbohydrate metabolism, is the body's primary fuel. It is used immediately for energy, or it is stored in the liver in the form of glycogen to be called upon at a later time. When the body is unable to metabolize carbohydrates, which are derived mainly from sugars and starches, the blood becomes overloaded with glucose. The kidneys are unable to handle the excess and in most cases it "spills" into the urine.

WHAT'S GONE WRONG?

If you have diabetes, something has gone awry in the elaborate system of metabolic checks and balances that the normal body uses to maintain a safe blood-sugar level. Sometimes the pancreas, a large gland located on the left side under the ribs, completely abdicates its job of turning out insulin, the hormone that helps the cells to use glucose as their fuel. Sometimes the pancreas secretes an inadequate amount of insulin, not enough to cope with the carbohydrates you eat. And sometimes the pancreas is unable to "recognize" the high blood-sugar level and so does not produce enough insulin in response to it even though the capacity is there.

In most cases, however, especially in older overweight diabetics, the pancreas continues to produce plenty of insulin, often much more than normal, but it can't perform its function of helping the cells use glucose. So plenty of insulin floats uselessly in the blood, unable to penetrate the cells, while sugar piles up but cannot be utilized.

The reason for this was once thought to be a deficient number of insulin receptors, but it is turning out to be more complex. One important factor seems to be the fat cell that we used to think was nothing but a stain on your shirt. In fact, it is a tiny factory that puts out twelve different substances, including adiponectin and resistin. Not producing enough adiponectin, which prevents diabetes, or putting out too much resistin, which resists the action of insulin, is probably what occurs in diabetics.

HOW DOES YOUR BODY MAKE INSULIN?

Insulin is manufactured by complicated little biochemical "factories" in the pancreas. These are the beta cells, responsible for so much of our well-being. They are located in the islets of Langerhans, one to two million tiny areas of the pancreas comprising maybe 2 percent of the entire gland.

The islets also secrete other hormones—glucagon from the alpha cells, somatostatin from the delta cells, and amylin from the beta cells, for example—which are deposited along with insulin, the main component, into the bloodstream via the tiny blood vessels that surround them. All of these hormones are involved in maintaining normal blood-sugar levels.

When it is working normally, the pancreas responds to every tiny fluctuation in blood sugar, releasing insulin whenever it is needed just as a thermostat turns a furnace off and on to maintain a constant temperature in your house. When the blood sugar rises after we eat, a signal goes to the pancreas, alerting it to move some insulin out.

When there is not enough glucose in the bloodstream to be used for fuel, the liver, stimulated by the glucagon from the islets' alpha cells, releases glucose from its warehouse of stored glycogen. At the same time, amylin alters the sensitivity and secretion of insulin and may help slow the absorption of sugar through the intestines. When a sufficient amount of glucose has been secreted by the liver, somatostatin is responsible for turning off the production before it goes too high.

It takes most people about two to three hours to return to the normal fasting blood-sugar level after a high-carbohydrate meal.

HOW IS INSULIN USED?

In the normal person, starches, sugars, and proteins (58 percent of which is eventually converted into carbohydrate) are broken down by the intestines into glucose, a form of sugar. The glucose is carried throughout the body by the bloodstream, entering the cells with the help of insulin, then burned for energy by the muscles. Some of the leftovers are stored in the muscle cells or converted into fat. The rest is stockpiled in the liver in the form of glycogen, to be called upon later if the blood sugar falls too low.

If there is not enough insulin or if the insulin available cannot help the glucose permeate the cells, this sugar accumulates in the blood, often in very high concentrations. The result is diabetes.

In a nondiabetic, glucose concentration is usually below 100 milligrams per 100 milliliters of blood plasma, and even after a huge overload of sugar rarely goes above 160 to 180 mgs. In uncontrolled diabetics, it can go much higher, frequently reaching 800 or even 1,000 mgs. Though there's obviously plenty of glucose available to feed the body's hungry tissues, it cannot be used effectively and the cells can literally starve, no matter how much you eat.

At the same time, the liver is stimulated to release its stores of sugar and then to begin a process called gluconeogenesis. In a response to an emergency call for more fuel, this important organ takes the huge amounts of amino acids produced by the starving tissues and changes them into more glucose. Fats are also transported to the liver. Now ketones, the end products of the burning of fat instead of carbohydrate for fuel, also overload the kidneys and spill into the urine. This is called ketoacidosis. When this happens, and nothing is done to remedy the situation, the body lapses into a diabetic coma—a real emergency.

By the way, people who are trying to lose weight on a high-fat diet such as Atkins also produce ketones, but this is not dangerous as long as their blood sugar remains normal. It is only when ketones are combined with high blood sugar that ketoacidosis becomes a problem.

TYPE 2 (NONINSULIN–DEPENDENT DIABETES MELLITUS, OR NIDDM)

About 92 percent of diabetics are type 2. If you are in this category, you continue to manufacture insulin, perhaps not enough to cover your needs, or perhaps more than enough, but it cannot be efficiently utilized. You can probably control your diabetes with diet and exercise, or diet combined with oral hypoglycemic drugs that stimulate the release of insulin, delay the absorption of carbohydrates, or lower your blood sugar by suppressing the liver's output of glucose. Or you may require insulin injections to supplement your own supply, or the new drugs called incretins to make your available insulin more effective.

Although your diabetes may have been discovered after you developed specific symptoms such as excessive thirst and urination, more likely you were diagnosed during a routine medical checkup. Or maybe your eye doctor or dentist was the first to suspect it. Most cases of type 2 occur gradually, and never present obvious warning signals.

Heredity plays a very important role for type 2s. We know there must be a genetic predisposition, perhaps resulting in early aging of the pancreatic cells or the shutdown of insulin receptors. When some kind of stress—overweight or pregnancy, for example—is added to the genetic tendency, diabetes is the result. The sumo wrestlers of Japan are programmed by their genes to gain tremendous amounts of weight. They are adored by the sportsmen of Japan, but develop diabetes and heart disease early in their lives. They blaze like meteors across the sky, but the trip is short.

The genetically isolated Pima Indians who live in a remote river valley in the Arizona desert tend to be sedentary, overweight, and diabetic. Half of the Pimas over thirty-five have diabetes, 15 times the incidence among the general population in the United States, the highest rate ever recorded. Yet those Pimas who live in Mexico and work the land usually remain thin and do not have evidence of increased diabetes.

Both groups are good examples of the inherited tendencies toward this disease combined with obesity. If you have a family history of diabetes, it would be extremely wise not to get fat.

Even teenagers may have this variety of diabetes (about 5 percent of type 2s are under twenty), more and more of them every year, but statistically it is probably likely to occur in people over forty, becoming more common by age fifty or sixty.

Eighty-five percent of type 2s have a diabetic parent, sibling, or other close relative. Those with an identical twin who is diagnosed with type 2 are almost certain to develop it, too, within a few years.

WHAT ARE THE CULPRITS?

The genetics of type 2 diabetes turns out to be very complicated, and the disease is thought to be caused, along with excess weight and a faulty lifestyle, by a variety of genes. A major development, reported in 2005, was the discovery of a variant gene—designated TCF7L2—that increases the risk of diabetes significantly and is thought to be carried by more than a third of the American population. According to the Iceland-based research team that identified it, people with one copy of the gene are estimated to have a 45 percent greater risk of type 2, while those who have inherited two copies, one from each parent, are 141 percent more likely to develop the disease.

The immediate practical effect of this discovery is that it may lead to diagnostic tests that can identify people with this gene, inspiring them to watch their weight, get plenty of exercise, and eat healthy diets.

Similar work goes on in many places. One study at the University of Texas Southwestern Medical Center has shown that a variation in the gene ENPPI is much more common in people with type 2 diabetes and those at greater risk for the disease. It may explain why certain ethnic groups have a higher risk even when they are thin. Changes in the gene PTPN1 are another possibility that may affect the production of a protein important in insulin activity. Variations in HNF4A, a gene that seems to act as a master regulator of insulin-making cells, seem to be much more common in type 2 diabetes. And Dr. C. Ronald Kahn of the Joslin Clinic has identified genes specifically involving PI3K that are defective in some type 2 diabetics.

What's more, type 2s are almost always overweight. The vast majority of adult diabetics are too heavy or even obese. Many overweight type 2s can lose their diabetes by losing weight. Sometimes a loss of even a few pounds is sufficient to accomplish this miracle because now you may produce enough of your own insulin to keep your blood sugar normal or decrease the visceral fat around your abdomen that interferes with the action of insulin.

In controlled studies, it has been discovered that regu-

lar, vigorous exercise can lower or even eliminate the
need for pills or injections.

Not all type 2 diabetes, however, is the result of overweight in a predisposed person. Sometimes it's simply
the result of an inefficient pancreas. The beta cells become unable to sense the sugar molecules and so can't
respond accurately to their presence; or they simply cannot produce enough insulin. In these cases, losing weight
won't help but eating correctly and enough exercising
will, perhaps supplemented by oral agents or insulin.

TYPE 1 (INSULIN-DEPENDENT DIABETES
MELLITUS, OR IDDM)

Type 1 diabetes, once known as juvenile diabetes, is
quite another story and may even be another disease
with a similar outcome. There are comparatively few
type 1s—less than 10 percent of the total number of diabetics.

Type 1 can strike at any age, and about 15 to 20 percent of IDDMs are adults when they are diagnosed. But
it happens for most people before they are twenty, and
most commonly around the ages of eight, twelve, and
puberty, when dramatic growth spurts take place. For
every 100,000 people in the country, there are 50 diagnosed diabetics under the age of five; there are 150 under
age ten; 270 below age fifteen; and 325 per 100,000 population by the age of eighteen.

Type 1 diabetes affects about one million Americans,
with about thirteen thousand new cases each year, making it the second largest childhood disease in the U.S.
after asthma.

It is now understood to be an autoimmune disease in

which a body's germ-fighting defenses mistakenly attack organs and tissues; in this case, the insulin-producing beta cells of the pancreas. Theory today is that the disease is usually triggered by a virus—perhaps a virus that is fairly benign for most people—that sets off an unrelenting immune response in a person who is genetically susceptible, knocking the beta cells permanently out of commission.

This kind of diabetes develops only in children and some adults who carry a very specific genetic make-up.

If you are a type 1, you have a marked insufficiency in the number of beta cells your pancreas possesses and you produce little or no insulin of your own. That means you must take insulin injections to compensate. Except in extremely rare cases, the oral drugs, designed to stimulate production in a pancreas that has the capability to make its own insulin, won't work for you.

Unlike type 2, type 1 diabetes generally shows up very abruptly and dramatically, with unmistakable symptoms—excessive urination and thirst, dramatic weight loss, weakness, irritability. If these symptoms go untreated, they rapidly progress into acidosis (see Chapter 9) and finally coma in only a few days or weeks.

As a type 1, a person with the severest form of diabetes, you probably do not have diabetic parents, though there is a genetic factor here, too, as studies with identical twins have shown. Far from overweight, you are probably very thin and perhaps wan. There is no way for you to lose your symptoms by losing weight and eating sanely. But supplementary insulin, aided by good diet and plenty of exercise, will keep your blood sugar relatively normal.

GENES PLAY A ROLE

Many genetic markers for type 1 diabetes have been identified only recently. If a child has genes HLA-DR3 or HLA-DR4 on his sixth chromosome, inherited from *both* parents, he has 2½ times more chance of becoming a type 1 diabetic after a viral infection. Eighty-five to 90 percent of all type 1 diabetics have DR3 and/or DR4. And if aspartic acid is not found in position 57 in these genes, the risk of diabetes increases even more. The worst-case scenario is to have both DR3 and DR4. But remember, even if a youngster has DR3 or DR4 genes, it is not inevitable that he or she will develop the disease.

Variants of another HLA gene may also play a role in this kind of diabetes. Researchers have recently found that DQA1 (0301) and DQB1 (0302), again on the sixth chromosome, are strong predictors of diabetes when passed along by two parents. Others—for example, DQB1 (0201) and DQB1 (0602)—are the most protective against it.

A second indicator is the presence of cytoplasmic pancreatic-islet-cell antibodies, found in 80 to 90 percent of children destined to become diabetics. In addition to these antibodies, the presence of genes ILA2 and GAD65 let us know when to start treatment. The likelihood of a child with all three indicators of becoming diabetic is almost 100 percent; with two of the three, it's 80 percent. Tests are currently under way at Columbia Presbyterean Medical Center in New York City to determine whether treating new-onset or recently diagnosed children with the antibody HOKT3Y (Ala-Ala) can preserve their beta cells.

But if, like the Inuits, a child has B7 on the sixth chromosome, his chances of diabetes are decreased. And if he has DR2, it is extremely doubtful he will get diabetes. Though people with DR2 make up a quarter of the population, only a few cases of diabetes have ever been reported among them.

Occasionally, diabetes is the result of another physical condition: pancreatitis, tumors, adrenal imbalance, injury to or removal of the pancreas, or damage caused by one of several drugs.

DOUBLE DOSE: TYPE 1½

Many people, perhaps 5 to 10 percent of all diabetics, do not fit neatly into the categories of type 1 or type 2. Instead, they have characteristics of both varieties. Like type 1, they harbor antibodies that attack the beta cells, reducing their insulin production to little or none. And like type 2, their disease develops slowly as they gradually lose their insulin-producing capability and eventually require insulin. They are usually overweight and have insulin resistance. The standard oral medications are usually not effective with this group, and they often need insulin to bring their sugar level down enough to ward off later complications.

DANGER: PREDIABETES

Prediabetics are people who have blood glucose levels that are higher than normal but not high enough to qualify them as true diabetics. With a fasting plasma glucose level between 100 mg/dl and 125 mg/dl, they have "impaired glucose tolerance" (IGT) and about half of them will be diagnosed as diabetics within ten years.

If you are in this category, you should be treated as a diabetic because you may already be on your way to its many unpleasant complications such as cardiovascular disease, kidney failure, and vision loss. You can lower your risk of continuing down the path to big trouble by losing weight (if you are too heavy), exercising regularly, cutting back on fats, eating judiciously (see Chapter 3), and maybe even taking an insulin-sensitizing medication (see Chapter 16 for more about stopping diabetes in its tracks).

WHO GETS DIABETES?

Diabetes gives geneticists headaches because it is almost impossible to predict, even in the presence of defective genes, who will eventually become diabetic, although many risk factors have recently been determined (see Chapter 16).

It was once thought that all the children of two diabetic parents would eventually become diabetic. Today it is thought that 60 percent is a more accurate figure. With one diabetic parent, sibling, or child, there is a 3 percent chance of diabetes by the age of forty to fifty-nine, a 10 percent chance after sixty.

The identical twin of a person who becomes diabetic before forty has a 30 percent likelihood of developing the disease. If the disease has its onset after forty, the chance an identical twin will have it increases to close to 100 percent, but if the disease does not occur within three years, the identical twin is probably home free. Fraternal twins, by the way, have about the same risk as other family members—about 10 percent.

EVERYTHING'S UNDER CONTROL

Diabetes is all about managing sugar. Once you know you are diabetic, you've got a new goal in life: to keep your blood sugar as close to normal as you possibly can. That means, ideally, between 70 mgs percent fasting and 150 mgs after a meal. That's not easy, especially in times of stress when every diabetic's blood sugar runs rampant, but you can stay within that range most of the time if you remember your future depends on it.

For many years, it was thought that this "tight control" was not too important as long as you felt well and functioned normally. Today we know differently.

GOOD CONTROL OR ELSE

Uncontrolled diabetes—consistently high blood sugars— can eventually affect every system of the body, resulting in many exotic varieties of diabetic complications. For example, people with diabetes are 2½ times more likely to suffer from strokes and 2 to 4 times more likely to develop cardiovascular disease. Over 60 percent of diabetics have high blood pressure and 60 to 70 percent have nerve disease. Diabetes is the leading cause of new cases of blindness in adults and of end-stage kidney disease. It is the primary cause of amputations, an estimated 82,000 of them in the U.S. in 2002. That's ten times the number of amputations for other reasons.

Those are frightening facts, but here's the good news: Control your diabetes—in other words, maintain your blood sugar at consistently normal levels—and you can avoid or minimize all of these nasty complications. A thirty-year study of 4,400 diabetics revealed that those people who had held their blood-sugar levels to below 300 mgs had three times less risk of complications after fifteen years of the disease than those with higher levels. Those with a level below 250 mgs had five to twenty times less risk. And those who kept their blood sugar below 120 on diet alone had almost no risk of complications at all.

In 1998, the United Kingdom Prospective Diabetes Study strongly proved and confirmed an earlier DCCT study that intensive treatment—be it with oral agents (sulfonylureas or metformin) or insulin—reduced diabetic complications equally but metformin seemed to be better for the heart. The study also showed reducing blood pressure greatly reduced complications.

In a study of the Pimas, it was found that complications occurred in the group with fasting sugars above 140 and above 200 two hours after eating. The higher the sugar, the more likely the complications, and follow-up data found that a long period of intensive control delayed the onset of complications for many years even when that control was later abandoned.

More recently, in December 2005, a long-awaited federally funded landmark study reported in the *New England Journal of Medicine* presented solid evidence that stringent blood sugar control can cut the risk of heart disease nearly in half, at least for type 1 diabetics. Type 2s are the subject of a similar large trial sponsored by the National Institutes of Health, with results expected in 2009.

NOBODY'S PERFECT

Of course, life is not fair. Some people who pay no attention to their control never develop complications in spite of their lack of vigilance, while others who exercise great care do get them in later years. But, in general, it is true that greater control means a better, healthier, longer life.

Nobody's perfect, and you won't be either. You will not always follow your diet plan, you will succumb to temptation now and then, you'll forget to test your blood sometimes, you will let your control get out of hand. But if this becomes your pattern and not just an occasional slip-up, you will undoubtedly pay the piper later. All the health problems associated with diabetes are hastened and exacerbated by poor control.

WHO'S IN CHARGE AROUND HERE?

You are. Your doctor will diagnose and prescribe and direct your treatment, but you are the only one who can live your own life. You're the one who puts the food into your mouth, decides how much exercise to get, takes the blood tests every day, handles the crises of hypoglycemia and high blood sugar. You can get direction and advice from your doctor and this book, but you are in charge of yourself.

This does not mean you are out there all on your own. It is very important that you see your doctor frequently, whether or not you take insulin. The doctor monitors your blood-sugar control in order to prevent complications in the future, picks up early changes, works with you on problems concerning diet, exercise, lifestyle, or whatever, and advises you on handling illnesses.

If you are a diabetic who is regulated by diet alone, see your doctor *at least* every three months. Don't go whenever you feel like it, or only when trouble brews. Go regularly on a scheduled basis.

If you take oral agents or insulin, make an appointment even more often, depending on your condition. Once every one to three months is right for most people. Never skip or postpone an appointment if you can possibly avoid it. And don't hesitate to call your physician if you see a change in the results of your home glucose monitoring.

To find a doctor who can give you good care, call your local chapter of the American Diabetes Association or the Juvenile Diabetes Foundation. You will be given the names of several doctors in your area who are the most knowledgeable about diabetes. This is a specialized field, and many general physicians are not qualified to handle your problems. Your future will be much brighter if you find a doctor who is.

IT'S A BALANCING ACT

Living with diabetes means a constant balancing act between the food you eat and the insulin you produce yourself or take by injection, along with the exercise you get. Insulin provides the mechanism for burning the food for energy to run your complex body. Exercise lowers your blood-sugar level. If you eat more food, you will need more insulin and exercise. If you eat less food, you will require less insulin and exercise. That's simple. What's hard is always having to think about this balancing act, especially at times when, often through no fault of your own, this balance is thrown out of kilter.

For many people, one of the most trying aspects is the need to be consistent, to lead a structured life. Especially if you take insulin, you soon discover that you must eat a preordained amount of carbohydrate, that you must eat on time, take your medication on schedule, take constant blood tests, check in with your doctor regularly. While everyone else, it seems, can stay up all night partying, eating pizza, and drinking sodas, stuffing themselves one day and fasting the next, paying no attention to medicines or doctors, you, if you are on NPH insulin, must plod along, day after day, on three meals plus two snacks.

That can be difficult, but it will pay off. Consistency isn't such a tremendous price to pay for feeling well now and in the future. It will eventually become a lifestyle you can live with.

2

MAKING THE DIAGNOSIS FOR DIABETES

To diagnose diabetes, your doctor must confirm through tests that you have inappropriately high blood sugar—sugar that rises to abnormal heights and stays there too long. In a nondiabetic, blood sugar rises and falls throughout the day, but never goes very high or very low because the pancreas secretes sufficient and efficient insulin.

HOW IS DIABETES DISCOVERED?

Many people are diagnosed as diabetic when urine or blood tests are made during routine examinations. Their symptoms are so minor that they don't even notice them. In fact, they may have had diabetes for years without knowing it. Other diabetics are discovered by their dentists who find unexplained periodontal problems, their podiatrists who spot suspicious foot sores, ophthalmologists who notice vision changes, other doctors who are looking for the underlying reasons for recurring vaginal or urinary infections, male sexual problems, menstrual irregularity, early menopause, itching (especially in the genital or anal areas), tingling, numbness, or fatigue.

THE OVERT SYMPTOMS

When diabetes occurs more suddenly or severely, the symptoms may be more sudden and severe, too. These include the three "polys": polyuria, polydipsia, and polyphagia.

Polyuria is excessive urination (when it occurs at night, it is known as excessive nocturia), and a strong sense of urgency. When the carbohydrate you eat is not utilized, it is dumped into the urine to be excreted from the body. Urine is produced in vast amounts, the bladder fills quickly, and much of an uncontrolled diabetic's time is spent in the bathroom. In babies, an increased need for diaper changes may be an indication of a problem.

The huge loss of water from the body tissues causes dehydration. Diabetics develop *polydipsia,* a tremendous thirst that can never be satisfied.

Polyphagia, excessive hunger, is the least common of the three major symptoms. It represents the body's frantic attempt to get the fuel it requires. Even though large amounts of food may be consumed, there will be rapid weight loss. One patient, a marine sergeant, was diagnosed after he continued to lose weight even though he ate one or two pounds of meat and drank two quarts of milk and juice with every meal.

Other symptoms of diabetes include weakness, heaviness of the legs so that climbing stairs or hills becomes extremely difficult, subnormal temperature, slow healing, dizziness, gum infections, tingling and loss of feeling in the hands or feet, acidosis, and, of course, diabetic coma.

Because uncontrolled diabetes is associated with an increased incidence of heart disease, blindness, miscarriage, and spontaneous abortion, these conditions may also raise in your doctor's mind the question of the possibility of diabetes.

JUST A MATTER OF ROUTINE

Discovering hyperglycemia—high blood sugar—with a urine test during a routine physical examination is a matter of chance if you are not severely diabetic. The urine must be checked at just the right moment. Glucose is carried in the bloodstream and travels through the kidneys. Below a blood-sugar level of about 156 mgs percent, most people will not lose sugar in the urine and it will not be discovered during the test. Instead, it will be returned to the body through the renal veins, which transport blood from the kidneys back to the heart. If you have a large meal but not enough insulin, or if it is not used effectively, some sugar will turn up in the urine. But this won't happen until an hour or so after the meal, when the food has had time to be turned into glucose and has made its way to the bladder from the kidneys via the bloodstream.

Even with excess blood sugar, a test taken an hour after a meal may be so diluted with urine accumulated *before* the meal that the sugar won't show up in concentrated amounts. Two to three hours after the meal, however, the urine will reflect the higher blood sugars.

The speed of the blood flow to the kidneys also influences how much sugar appears in the urine. Sometimes, especially with diseases like heart failure, this rate drops, and, even though the sugar is high, even far above 156 mgs, very little escapes into the urine. The doctor making the diagnostic tests should take this high renal threshold into account.

In pregnancy, the reverse happens and there is an increased rate of blood flow to the kidneys. Now more sugar appears in the urine at *lower* levels. That means all pregnant women with sugar in the urine are not necessarily diabetic, though they should definitely be tested for the possibility.

MAKING THE DIAGNOSIS FOR DIABETES

For many years the gold standard for the diagnosis of diabetes was the glucose tolerance test (GTT), which we will describe later, but it is gradually being replaced by a simpler, less expensive, and less time-consuming procedure, the fasting plasma glucose test.

THE FASTING PLASMA GLUCOSE TEST

This test, now deemed sufficient for diagnosis by the American Diabetes Association, requires a sample of blood taken from your arm after you have had nothing but water for at least the previous eight hours. Your sugar level should be no higher than 126 mgs percent to be considered normal, or 140 mgs percent in pregnancy.

Sometimes another procedure is added: the two-hour postprandial plasma glucose test, when your blood sugar is measured two hours after consuming 75 grams of carbohydrates. If it is over 200 mgs percent, you will be classified as diabetic.

HbA1c: THE LAST WORD

The purpose of an HbA1c (glycohemoglobin) test is to monitor blood-glucose control and it is not yet widely used for diagnosing diabetes, but you can be fairly sure you have diabetes if this test comes up with a higher-than-normal result. The HbA1c, a blood assay that requires only one blood sample taken at any time, no matter when you last ate, measures your level of glycated hemoglobin and reflects an average of your blood-sugar levels over the last two or three months.

Hemoglobin, a protein in red blood cells that carries oxygen to the body's cells, attaches to glucose in the bloodstream when glucose is elevated and stays attached for the life of the blood cell, about 120 days. It is this glycated hemoglobin that can be measured. If you have a glycated hemoglobin level of 6.2 percent or more (the norm in most laboratories is 3.2 to 6.2 percent), you can be classified as a diabetic, even without an official glucose tolerance test. The minimum level of 6.2 percent may be changed to 5.3 percent in the near future because it reflects a more realistic value and should be your goal. When you get your report from the laboratory, remember that only the A1c value is relevant (some labs report other components as well).

The relationship of mean blood glucose (MBG) to A1c may be explained this way: MBG equals 30.9 glycohemoglobin (GHB) minus 60.6. In other words, every 1 percent change in GHB is associated with a blood glucose change of 31 mgs/dl. At 7 percent the average blood glucose is 155.7 mgs/dl, and at 9 percent is 217.5 mgs/dl.

THE GLUCOSE TOLERANCE TEST

Here's how the glucose tolerance test is done:

Before you have a glucose tolerance test, you *must* eat at least 100 to 150 grams of carbohydrate a day for at least *three* days. This is, for most people, a normal amount. If you have been eating very little carbohydrate, the glucose tolerance test will catch your pancreas unawares and the results may not be accurate.

Diuretics and estrogen supplements may also influence a glucose tolerance test interpretation. The test is best done in the morning, sitting down and relaxed. No smoking until it is completed.

On the morning of the test, you are asked to eat no breakfast. Your first blood sample will reflect a *fasting* state—no incoming food for at least the previous eight hours. The doctor or laboratory technician will draw a tube of blood from your arm, then give you a drink of quickly absorbed glucose. This must be swallowed within five minutes. An hour later another blood sample is drawn, followed by samples taken at two hours and three hours (and sometimes at four and five hours). The glucose content of each blood sample is carefully measured.

WHAT THE BLOOD TELLS US

The glucose tolerance test gives readings of blood sugar for at least four different time periods—fasting, one hour, two hours, three hours. These are plotted into a curve and analyzed.

For the normal person without diabetes or hypoglycemia, blood sugar throughout the day will be between 0.070 and 0.2 grams per 100 cc of blood. In other words, whether or not you have recently had a meal, there is always approximately 7 to 20 parts sugar to one hundred parts of blood. A whole-blood value of 70 to 100 mgs percent corresponds to a blood *serum* level of 115 mgs percent. The serum, the fluid left after the blood cells and blood-clotting substances are removed, is what is tested in virtually all chemical determinations today.

A few home monitors measure whole blood, which has lower sugar content for the same volume than serum alone, but commerical laboratories and almost all home monitors today measure serum.

In the normal person, the serum level rises an hour after eating to no more than 175 mgs percent (up to 200 mgs is still considered normal), and at two hours drops back to no more than 140 mgs percent. At three hours, it returns to the fasting level.

But, if you are a diabetic, your numbers will be different. When your fasting level is above 125 mgs, your one-hour level above 175 mgs, two-hour level above 145, and three-hour level above 125, you have abnormally elevated glucose and you have confirmed diabetes.

Sometimes a diagnosis is made when three out of the four tests on the curve show elevated glucose, and sometimes a system of totaling the numbers is used. When the fasting, one-hour, two-hour, and three-hour results are added together and produce a sum below 500, you are considered normal. From 500 to 800, you may be diabetic. With a total over 800, you are definitely diabetic.

Treatment—diet alone, or diet plus oral agents or insulin—is necessary if you have the symptoms of diabetes as well as abnormal sugars, or if you have no symptoms but have a fasting sugar over 126 and a two-hour sugar over 200.

The following chart gives examples of representative glucose tolerance tests:

TYPICAL GLUCOSE TOLERANCE TEST RESULTS

	Fasting	*1 hour*	*2 hours*	*3 hours*	*4 hours*	*5 hours*
Normal glucose	80 mgs	125 mgs	90 mgs	86 mgs	84 mgs	86 mgs
Type 2 Diabetic (NIDDM)	150	230	210	150	118	—
Type 1 Diabetic (IDDM)	250	440	300	280	250	200

GUIDELINES FOR DIABETES DIAGNOSIS

In 2005, the blood-sugar levels traditionally used to diagnose diabetes were reviewed and revised downward by the American Diabetes Association and endorsed by federal health authorities. A blood-sugar level below 140 mgs percent used to be considered normal. Now, if you have a sugar level over 126 milligrams per deciliter, in two readings, on two different days, on a fasting plasma glucose test, you are classified as diabetic.

The new criteria were developed after it was shown that 10 to 20 percent of diabetic patients develop complications such as eye, kidney, and blood-vessel damage by the time their glucose level reaches 126 mgs percent. With earlier detection and treatment, these complications could be delayed or even prevented.

Here are the new numbers:

A normal fasting blood-sugar level is 100 mgs percent or less. Prediabetes (impaired glucose tolerance or IGT), is defined as 100 to 126 mgs percent. And diabetes is confirmed with blood sugar over 126 mgs percent.

At two hours after eating, 140 mgs percent or less is deemed normal; 140 to 199 mgs is prediabetes or IGT; 200 mgs percent or higher is classified as diabetes.

HIGH SUGAR AND YOUR HEART

Diabetes is a powerful risk factor for heart disease and stroke. In a study of almost 7,000 healthy men, ages forty-four to fifty-five, enrolled in the Paris Prospective Study from 1968 and 1973 and followed up for twenty-three years, it was found that the death rate from coronary heart disease almost doubled among those volunteers with fasting blood sugars consistently over 124 mgs. The rate tripled for the men with sugars over 140.

Translation: the higher your sugar level, the higher your chances of developing heart disease. See Chapter 10 for more bad news.

ALMOST DIABETES BUT NOT QUITE

Sometimes blood tests reveal that you are not actually a diabetic but a prediabetic, someone who is almost surely going to get the real thing if you don't watch out. Prediabetes is a condition, also called impaired glucose tolerance, or IGT, that means your fasting blood-sugar levels are between 100 and 126 mg/dl, higher than normal but not high enough to be considered diabetes. You are somewhere between the normal healthy person and the diabetic, perhaps with your blood sugar becoming abnormally elevated in response to glucose, then returning almost to normal after three hours.

If you are prediabetic, you do not have diabetes. On the other hand, you will probably develop it within ten years if you don't take action. Seven percent of those with confirmed prediabetes or IGT convert to the real thing every year, and half eventually end up with it. See Chapter 16 for more information.

If this is your diagnosis, you must see your doctor for tests at least once a year and perhaps even start treatment. You will need a glucose tolerance test and an A1c test. If your A1c results are 5.3 mgs or higher or your fasting blood sugar is between 100 and 126 mgs, you should be treated as a diabetic. Changes in lifestyle—losing weight, eating properly, and getting more exercise—are the first step. If they don't get your blood sugar down into the normal range, then medication may do the job.

3

NOBODY LOVES A DIET

Ask 100 people to tell you the secret of diabetes control and 99 of them will answer "insulin." They are wrong. The real secret lies not in that little white bottle, or even in small white, blue, or yellow pills, but in your refrigerator and kitchen cabinets. That fact is not glamorous, mysterious, or even very interesting, but it is true.

What you eat—your diet—is the single most important key to diabetic control. It is the best blood-sugar-lowering agent, the most effective and the least expensive. With diet, plus a certain amount of physical activity, you may not need insulin or oral antidiabetic agents at all. The vast majority of type 2 diabetics can be controlled with diet alone. Many diabetics who now take oral agents or insulin won't need them anymore if they eat correctly. And some who are overweight will lose all their diabetic symptoms *completely* simply by taking off a few pounds.

As for those diabetics who have truly deficient pancreases and therefore require insulin injections to supply their bodies with this essential hormone, and for those who can never utilize their own insulin efficiently without the help of oral agents, diet is *still* the most important ingredient of treatment. Diabetics can never achieve good control, with or without medication, unless they eat correctly.

Nobody loves a diet. Diets tell you not to eat this, and that you must eat that—no fun at all. Most people, when they are first diagnosed as diabetics, are concerned about the need to change their eating habits. After all, the majority of diabetics are overweight and they love food. They don't want to think about every bite that goes into their mouths.

But we are going to make it simple by prescribing what we believe to be the world's easiest and most effective diet. Never have diabetics had to think less about their food than with this plan. And yet it works.

This diet is not concerned with calories (unless, of course, you want to lose weight). It is concerned only with carbohydrates. *You must eat no more than a certain number of grams of carbohydrates (though not refined sugar) at every meal. That is the only rule. Aside from that, you can eat anything you like if your weight is where you want it to be.*

The diet presented here will not make you miserable, frustrated, or confused. It will keep your blood sugar within the normal range that is now your chief goal. It is safe. It can be followed for a lifetime without difficulty. You won't feel deprived. It is good not only for you, but for the rest of your family as well, so it doesn't require preparing separate meals. As you can see, with only a little caution you can eat just like the rest of the world.

THE CHANGING SCENE IN DIABETIC DIETS

Before the discovery of insulin in 1922, a harsh dietary regimen was the only treatment for diabetes. It usually included very little carbohydrate because once the blood sugar went up it would take off like a runaway train, precipitating a hasty demise as a result of diabetic coma.

Diabetics were placed on starvation diets so low in calories that growth was retarded and they died of malnutrition if not diabetic complications. Or they were given diets that included only milk and barley water boiled with bread; or rancid meats, fat, and milk served up with lime water, cathartics, and opium; or fat combined with alcohol and vegetables boiled three times before they could be eaten. One nineteenth-century physician made sure his patients ate exactly what he prescribed by locking them in their rooms and opening their doors only to offer them their meager meals.

Once insulin was discovered, many doctors decided that patients taking injections could eat whatever they liked, which proved to be a mistake. Others still insisted that carbohydrates be kept low, perhaps to about 30 percent of the daily intake, with the major part of the calories made up of protein and fat.

Now we know, however, that diabetics—who already have an accelerated tendency toward arteriosclerosis, heart attacks, and strokes—were hastened along the road to vascular disease by the high-fat diet. The diet, in other words, was probably killing more people than it helped. In the early seventies, the American Diabetes Association recommended that diabetics eat the same proportion of carbohydrates as most other people do— 50 percent or more.

But even with the liberalizing of the diet, many people continue to find it extremely difficult to stay with a plan that is rigid or complicated. The diet you'll find here is easy to live with, simple, rational, logical. Besides, it works wherever you are. You can follow it to achieve normal blood sugar whether you eat at home, in restaurants, or traveling around the world.

THE WORLD'S EASIEST DIABETIC DIET

To follow this diet, there is just one rule: *avoid simple carbohydrates such as sugar, honey, and syrups and eat 40 to 45 grams of complex carbohydrates at every meal.* (Exception: If you are engaging in strenuous exercise, you may need more.)

Forty to 45 grams of carbohydrate amounts to 50 to 60 percent of your daily food, approximating the typical American diet. The rest of your menu will include protein, fats, and water in whatever proportions you choose. If you are not trying to reduce, you may eat as much of these foods as you wish. If you are, you can control your calories up or down simply by adjusting your meat portions. Or, if you prefer, you may incorporate the food exchange lists of the American Diabetes Association to help you keep your calories counted.

Most diets designed for diabetics not only place greater emphasis on cutting back carbohydrates (usually cutting them back too much), but also regulate the amount of proteins and fats you can eat at each meal. However, unless you are among the very small number of people whose control is very precarious (there are some slim people who are uncontrolled on diet or oral agents who, with a restricted calorie diet, may avoid insulin) or you are trying to lose weight, there is no need to be concerned about anything but your carbohydrate intake. You will probably consume about the same amounts of proteins and fats every day anyway, and even if you stray from your usual habits one day it won't disturb your blood sugar enough to cause problems when you are in good control.

So, simply keep tabs on your carbohydrates. And relax!

WHAT'S IN FOOD?

All foods are made up of carbohydrate, protein, or fat, plus water, minerals, vitamins, and fiber.

Carbohydrates (found mainly in sugar, starch, fruits, and vegetables) are the natural fuel of the body and supply the energy to run all its complicated systems. If there is a shortage of carbohydrates in your diet, you will start burning fat, which, in a diabetic, can lead to serious problems. Together with protein and fats, carbohydrates promote the growth and maintenance of body cells. Every gram of carbohydrate is equal to 4 calories.

Proteins are the building blocks of the body, needed for growth and repair of body tissues. Most protein foods (chiefly meat, milk, cheese, eggs, fish) contain a large proportion of fat as well. Approximately 58 percent of the protein we eat is slowly converted to carbohydrate. Each gram of protein is equal to 4 calories.

Fats provide a concentrated source of energy and add flavor to foods. They carry vitamins along with essential fatty acids, and provide cushioning for vital organs. Each gram of fat equals 9 calories. About 10 percent of the fat we eat is converted to carbohydrate.

Water is needed for all the digestive processes and is an essential part of all tissues.

Minerals and iron promote strong bones and teeth, healthy circulatory, muscular, and nervous systems, blood hemoglobin, etc.

Vitamins are essential for the proper functioning of all systems of the body.

Fiber (or roughage) is not a nutrient, but important for efficient digestion and, it is thought, helps maintain normal blood-sugar levels.

WHAT IS A CALORIE?

A calorie is the amount of energy required to raise the temperature of 4 gallons of water one degree Farenheit. Another way of putting it is that it is the energy expended by a seated man turning a doorknob.

Though most diets are based on calorie-counting, we are not concerned here with calories—unless, of course, you want to lose weight. Then calories definitely do count because weight cannot be lost (except *temporarily* through water loss on high-protein diets) without cutting calories.

WHY THINK ABOUT GRAMS?

It's all a numbers game. Our diet uses grams as the basic weight measurement of food. Why? Because grams are much easier to count and manipulate than ounces and pounds, and much more exact. (One pound equals 456 grams, while 1 ounce equals 30 grams. A nickel weighs 5 grams.)

It is essential for our diet to know the number of grams of carbohydrate in each food. That's because we must know how much of that food will enter the bloodstream in the form of sugar, and how quickly it will be absorbed. A diabetic can safely handle only a certain amount of sugar at one time. Too much too fast will raise a diabetic's blood sugar too high too quickly.

Every food can be analyzed into grams of carbohydrate, protein, and fat. For example, a standard slice of bread weighs about 1 ounce, or 30 grams. This slice of bread contains 15 grams of carbohydrate, 2½ grams of protein, and 12½ grams of nondigestible material and water.

A small orange weighing 100 grams contains about 10 grams of carbohydrate.

Thirty grams (1 ounce) of meat has no carbohydrate, 7 grams of protein, and 5 grams of fat. The rest is non-digestible material.

WHY CONCENTRATE ON CARBOHYDRATES?

You must know how much sugar is entering your blood-stream at any one time, because this is the main influence on your blood-sugar level. You require a certain amount, which is derived from carbohydrate, for your brain and body to function, but you cannot cope with too much. So it's a matter of portion control when it comes to carbohydrates. You can probably cope with 3 ounces of orange juice, but 8 ounces will send your blood sugar off the wall.

The normal fate of 100 grams of carbohydrate eaten at one sitting is as follows: 25 grams are used by the brain and red blood cells; 60 grams are delivered to the liver to be stored as glycogen for later release or transported into the fatty-acid cycle; the remaining 15 grams are rationed out via the bloodstream to the periphery of the body to be used by the muscles at a rate of 5 grams an hour.

In the nondiabetic, this balance is always maintained by the prompt response of the pancreas to rising blood sugar. But diabetics are different. Because you produce insufficient insulin or your cells cannot absorb the glucose readily, your blood-sugar levels are not kept at the normal percentage but can rise astronomically when too much carbohydrate is eaten at one time. And they can remain high for a very long time. The excess glucose is excreted along with the urine, or it stays in the blood-stream as elevated blood sugar.

THE NITTY-GRITTY OF CARBOHYDRATES

Carbohydrates contain one or more chains of 3 to 7 carbons, 12 hydrogens, and 6 oxygens, bound together. The smaller the number of chains, the faster they are absorbed by the body.

One-chain carbohydrates are monosaccharides, such as glucose, fructose, and galactose. These are absorbed into the bloodstream very quickly.

Oligosaccharides are usually composed of two to four or more chains of simple sugars, the best known being sucrose found in cane sugar and beets, maltose found in starch, and lactose in milk.

Polysaccharides are long and complex chains of sugar that are the readily digestible storage materials of plant and animal cells. These are starch, dextrin, and glycogen. They are more slowly absorbed and have less immediate effect on blood sugar.

Sorbitol and mannitol are "sugar alcohols," frequently ingredients of "dietetic" foods. About 50 percent turns into sugar but it is absorbed slowly and the small amounts in sugarless gum or mints don't add up to enough to affect your blood sugar unless, of course, you eat too much of them. You'd find that twelve pieces of sorbitol-sweetened hard candy, for example, would affect your blood sugar. Besides, twelve pieces would contain 150 calories and might cause diarrhea.

WHAT YOU CAN'T EAT

Foods that contain simple carbohydrates or sugars—the monosaccharides—must be avoided except upon rare occasions. They contain many calories but very little nutrition. More important, they are *much* too quickly absorbed by the bloodstream. They are too potent. They are

available too soon, too precipitously, to be effectively handled by diabetics, especially if you take insulin. They are
dangerous for you (except when you *need* them to raise
your blood sugar in a hurry). DO NOT EAT THEM.

Foods containing simple carbohydrates or sugars include:

Candy

Cereals that are sugar-coated
or contain sweetening

Condensed milk

Dried fruits

Honey

Jams and jellies

Marmalade and preserves

Molasses

Pastries and cookies

Puddings, pies, and cakes

Raisins

Regular chewing gum

Regular soft drinks

Sugar, any variety, any color

Sweet wine

Syrups

Other foods that diabetics should avoid because they
raise blood-sugar levels far too fast (except if you are
having an insulin reaction) are:

Apple juice

Apples

Gatorade

Gelatin desserts (regular)

Grape juice

Instant breakfasts or
"diet" bars

Maple-sugar-flavored bacon
or sausage

Pineapple

Pineapple juice

Processed yogurt with
fruit or flavoring (most
brands)

Prune juice

Sherbet

Yams and sweet potatoes

Sometimes you can be surprised by the foods that
tend to raise your blood sugar too fast. For example,
some people can tolerate ice cream more easily than
potatoes. Dietetic pies may be made without added
sugar but the fruit in them contains sugar and their
crusts must be counted as carbohydrates. Even sugar-

free jams and jellies contain natural sugars. An occasional smear isn't a problem but in normal amounts they raise your blood sugar too much.

There has been a lot of talk about the "glycemic index," which means that some foods have more effect on your blood sugar than others even though they may be equivalent in carbohydrate content. You can determine what your glycemic index is for particular foods by testing your blood two hours after you eat them, taking into account the other foods eaten in the same meal. This is easy if you have a glucose meter. If you find that a certain food sends your blood sugar sky high, avoid it or simply eat less of it.

IS SUGAR ABSOLUTELY OFF-LIMITS?

Diabetics have long been told to stay away from sugar and sugar-laden foods because simple carbohydrates cause a sudden surge in blood glucose levels, and we are telling you that very same thing again right here. Despite what you may have been reading recently, simple sugars are more quickly absorbed into the bloodstream than other carbohydrates such as starches or complex carbohydrates.

If you yearn for something sweet, it won't hurt you to substitute a cookie or two, a piece of pound cake, or a scoop of ice cream once in a great while for an *equal* amount of carbohydrate in your meal plan. Just remember, however, that you're not getting the same nutrition from a cookie as, say, an orange. And a chocolate peanut chew is certainly not better for you than a couple of slices of bread unless at that very moment you are overdosing on insulin.

By the way, many people think that sugar-free cookies are perfectly safe, but they forget that although these cookies contain no sugar, they are made with starch, which is carbohydrate. So they must be counted as carbohydrates. Read the box to find out how much. The same goes for "dietetic" pies. After all, they have crusts made with flour, a carbohydrate, and they contain fruit, more carbohydrate, so watch out.

WHAT YOU CAN EAT: THE COMPLEX CARBOHYDRATES

The complex carbohydrates, some of the oligosaccharides and the polysaccharides, are the ones that must make up most of your 40 to 50 grams per meal. They are a much better source of energy than fatty foods because they have less than half the calories of fat and the same amount as protein, and often contain more nutrition in the form of vitamins, minerals, and fiber. Besides, they can make you feel full and more satisfied.

The complex carbohydrates include grains, starches, some vegetables, and legumes. They are absorbed much more slowly than the simple carbohydrates and, eaten in certain amounts, won't raise your blood sugar to abnormal heights that may overwhelm your body. If you stay within the guidelines, your blood sugar should measure no more than 126 mgs percent fasting and 199 mgs percent two hours after a meal—just where we want it.

If you find that this is not true for you, then you must make adjustments in the food you eat. Nothing is chiseled in stone and everything can be changed to suit your special needs. Half a white potato, for example, would be bad for some people, but it may not be bad for you. Check it out by testing your blood sugar two hours after you eat it.

For your 40 to 45 grams of carbohydrates per meal, choose from the food lists that follow: 10-gram fruits and desserts; 15-gram starches; 3-percent vegetables; 6-percent vegetables.

Each meal should include no more than 2 units from the 15-gram list (the equivalent of 2 slices of bread) unless you're about to engage in heavy physical activity, in which case you'll need more. You need this slowly absorbed carbohydrate to carry you over to your next meal or snack. Fruits and juices, because they are so quickly digested and absorbed, raising your blood sugar more rapidly, *cannot be used as most or all of your total allotment.*

Keep your meals well balanced and varied, and eat the rest of your calories in proteins and fats as you like. How much of these you eat is a matter of taste and habit. Most people consume about the same amounts every day or every week. If, however, you are watching your weight or your cholesterol level, then your proteins and fats should be limited, as we will discuss a little later.

Diabetics who take insulin must take care to eat the *same* amount of food, including the *right* amount of carbohydrate, every day, spaced out in the *same* way, because your insulin dose is based on the food you consume.

If, however, you are now taking the newer insulins, you've got a lot more freedom. Suppose, for example, you take Lantus at night and Humalog, Novolog, or Apidra (or the oral agents Prandin or Starlix) just before meals. Because you don't take the quick-acting insulin until you're ready to eat and you won't have the "peaks" you have on the older long-acting insulins, you can be much more relaxed about eating on time. In fact, you could even skip a meal, something that has always been strictly forbidden. It is, however, still preferable for diabetics not to skip meals and to eat three times a day.

NOTE: You will see that we have included milk and plain yogurt in *both* the 10-gram (fruits) list and the

15-gram (starches) list. Because they are intermediate in both absorption rate and carbohydrate content, you may substitute them for foods on either list. They also contain protein and fat. Avoid the flavored and fruited yogurts. Vanilla yogurt, for example, has twice as much carbohydrate as plain. Some brands of cherry yogurt have almost three times as much. Always check the container for carbohydrate content and figure it into your total amount for that meal.

Tomato sauce is also on two lists, the 10-gram list and the 6-percent vegetable list, because its carbohydrate content falls between the two.

Foods containing 10 grams of carbohydrate

2 medium apricots	1 small peach
½ medium banana	1 small pear
½ cup blueberries, black-berries, or raspberries	2 small plums
	2 cups popcorn
½ small cantaloupe	1 cup strawberries
9 cherries	1 large tangerine
6 ounces diet cranberry juice	8 ounces (1 cup) tomato juice or 6 ounces vegetable juice
¼ cup diet cranberry sauce	
1 medium fresh fig	½ cup tomato sauce
½ medium grapefruit	1 cup watermelon balls
5 ounces grapefruit juice	¾ cup plain yogurt
15 grapes	1 scoop ice cream*
3 medium lemons	1 scoop ice milk*
½ small mango	1 scoop frozen yogurt
⅛ large melon (honeydew)	½ cup evaporated milk
1 medium nectarine	8 ounces (1 cup) milk†
1 small orange	
3 ounces orange juice	

---

* Vanilla, chocolate, coffee, or strawberry. If you eat dietetic ice cream, you may have ¼ pint, the equivalent of a 10-gram serving.
† Whole, skim, low-fat, buttermilk, or powdered (¼ cup diluted with ¾ cup water).

Also:

5 animal crackers
1 "thin" slice of bread
1 slice protein bread
2 fortune cookies
3 gingersnaps
44 thin pretzel sticks
2 graham crackers
2 Lorna Doones

18 oyster crackers
5 Ritz crackers
4 Saltines
3 Social Teas
3 Triscuits
2 Uneeda Biscuits
8 Wheat Thins

Foods containing 15 grams of carbohydrate

1 slice bread (white, rye, pumpernickel, whole wheat, French, Italian)
1 small plain roll
½ hamburger roll
1 hot-dog roll
½ large pita
½ slice pizza
½ matzoh
4 small matzoh balls
1 small plain muffin or biscuit
¼ medium bagel
½ plain doughnut
½ English muffin
½ plain croissant
1 slice French toast (without sugar)
1 cheeze blintz
5 thin Melba toasts
3 Zwieback toasts
2 bread sticks
15 potato chips
1 5-inch waffle
1 4-inch pancake
1 small corn muffin
1 8-inch tortilla
2 6-inch taco shells
¼ cup bread crumbs
1 piece marble or pound

cake (same weight as 1 slice of bread) on special occasions
3 dietetic chocolate chip cookies

Also:

½ cup cooked rice, barley, groats, grits
½ cup cooked macaroni, spaghetti, or other pasta
½ cup cooked egg noodles
1 medium white potato
½ cup mashed potatoes
7½ medium French fries
⅓ cup cooked dry beans (lentil, mung, pinto, red, black, etc.)
¼ cup cooked soybeans
½ small ear corn or ⅓ cup kernels
½ cup cooked cereal
½ cup bran cereal (no raisins)
1 cup puffed cold cereal
¾ cup most other cold cereals
2 tbsp. wheat germ (plain)

2 tbsp. miller's bran	*Also:*
1 small California avocado or ½ small Florida avocado	8 ounces (1 cup) milk* ½ cup evaporated milk 1 cup plain yogurt

NOTE: Any item from the 10-gram list becomes 15 grams by taking one and a half portions. Be careful, however, when you consume more fruit, because it may be absorbed so quickly that it will raise your blood sugar too high and too fast. The only way to check its effect on you is to make frequent blood tests soon after you've eaten it.

Water-packed canned fruits may be eaten in the same amounts as fresh fruit. For example, remember that two halves of a canned pear equal 1 small pear. Don't eat more.

Beware of soup! Sometimes—especially for people who produce little of their own insulin—a bowl of vegetable, lentil, or bean soup will make their blood sugars soar. That's because when legumes are cooked, their skins are softened and their carbohydrate is made available to be absorbed directly into the bloodstream instead of going through the bowel. Our advice: Stay away from soups you can't see through (gazpacho is the only exception we can think of). Again, you can find out if this applies to you by monitoring your blood sugar soon after you've eaten opaque soup.

You may have noticed that sweet potatoes are not on the list of permissible foods. However, if you really love them, you may have half a medium potato *if* you don't eat your other carbohydrates at the same meal, and *if* you check your blood sugar two hours after eating them and find that it falls within the acceptable range.

---

* Whole, skim, low-fat, buttermilk, or powdered (¼ cup diluted with ¾ cup water).

Another note: Find out where your avocados come from. A small rough-skinned California avocado usually contains only 6.5 grams of carbohydrate while a small smooth-skinned Florida avocado may have up to 13 grams.

A VERITABLE VARIETY OF VEGETABLES

Vegetables also contain carbohydrate, and it is important to know how much of them you can safely eat. The following list includes those that have only 3 grams of carbohydrate per 100 grams of weight and in most cases influence your blood sugar very little. They consist mainly of water and nondigestible fiber. Eat them as raw as you like. If cooked, limit them to about 1 cup per portion.

3-percent vegetables

Asparagus, fresh
Bamboo shoots
Bean sprouts
Broccoli
Cabbage
Cauliflower
Celery
Cucumber
Eggplant
Endive
Green or wax beans
Green peppers
Kohlrabi
Lettuce, romaine, chicory, escarole
Mushrooms
Parsley
Radishes
Rhubarb (no sugar)
Sauerkraut
Spinach
Summer squash
Swiss chard
Turnips
Watercress
Zucchini

The 6-percent vegetables have 6 grams of carbohydrate for every 100 grams of weight and cannot be taken ad lib by many diabetics. These are usually restricted to ½ cup per meal (or counted as 5 grams of your total of 40 to 45 grams). If you want to eat more, subtract appropriately from your starch.

6-percent vegetables

Artichokes   Pumpkin
Brussels sprouts   Red peppers
Carrots   Tomatoes
Green peas   Tomato sauce
Kale   Turnips
Okra   Winter squash
Onions, leeks, chives,
   scallions

THE SECRET OF SUCCESS

The only way you can successfully stick to the 40 to 45 grams per meal of carbohydrate without constantly counting and figuring and going bananas is to remember the equivalent of *two slices of bread!*

Once you can remember that the equivalent (which is how much *complex* carbohydrate you must have every meal—30 grams) is 1 cup of rice or pasta, 2 medium potatoes, 15 French fries, 1 English muffin, ⅔ cup of corn, 1 cup of cooked cereal, etc., you can go anywhere, eat in any restaurant and be perfectly safe. We are assuming you will not only eat your two-slices-of-bread equivalent per meal but another 10 to 20 grams of carbohydrate as well.

Your body cannot distinguish between rice or bread or beans. Or, from the fruit list, it doesn't know the difference between strawberries, grapefruit, or blueberries. It only knows it is getting so many grams of complex or simple carbohydrates. Interchange the foods on each list as you like and your body won't care.

By the way, pasta cooked *al dente* contains more carbohydrate than well-cooked pasta because it has less water content (the longer it cooks, the more water it absorbs), so your portion should be a little smaller. The sauce on your pasta makes a difference as well. Sauces such as garlic and olive oil, primavera, and pesto are acceptable, but watch out for tomato sauce. Tomato sauce raises blood sugar too quickly for most diabetics, especially those on insulin.

PLANNING YOUR MEALS

To plan meals, there is only one rule: *40 to 45 grams of carbohydrate, with at least 30 grams coming from the starch list.* There's no need to count right down to the very last gram—*approximately* 40 to 45 is sufficient. This makes it very simple. If you can remember the national anthem, you will soon remember the values of the foods you usually eat.

Do not save carbohydrates from one meal to another. Eat your full allotment at each meal or you may run into low-sugar trouble.

Eat about the same number of grams of carbohydrate every day (the only exception: when you plan unusually heavy exercise or nonexercise. See Chapter 4). This is most important for insulin-users, not so critical for those on oral agents, and usually matters not at all if you are diet-controlled. But dosages of insulin are designed to correspond to your food intake. If your carbohydrate intake changes, you will suffer from too much insulin or too little.

Let's start with breakfast.

BREAKFAST

We will assume you eat the typical American breakfast, but you may make your own choices as long as you avoid simple sugars and limit yourself to 40 to 45 grams of other carbohydrates. You only need to do your arithmetic.

For example, you might choose one of the following:

- 3 ounces orange juice, 8 ounces tomato juice, or ½ cantaloupe for your breakfast fruit. This accounts for 10 grams of carbohydrate.

Then, adding another 30 grams, choose among these:

- 2 slices toast, 2 halves English muffin, ½ bagel, 2 small corn muffins, 2 4-inch pancakes, or 2 slices of French toast. These are worth 15 grams each or 30 grams in all.
- Coffee or tea.

This meal contains about 40 grams of carbohydrate.

If you prefer cereal, have 1 cup of cold cereal with 8 ounces of milk or 1 cup of hot cereal with 4 ounces of milk.

HELPFUL HINTS

Sometimes you may want ½ banana on your cereal. Then omit the juice or other fruit, or drink only a small glass of tomato juice.

If you'd like to add eggs or bacon or any other protein or fat, feel free. The only reason to restrict them is for weight or cholesterol reduction.

Why can't you eat a whole bagel as your 30 grams of bread? Because a bagel is the equivalent of four slices of bread (60 grams). Your portion is half a bagel, even if you've scooped out some of the middle. Think of it this way: if you threw a bagel at somebody's head you could kill him but if you threw two slices of bread at him he'd laugh. Bagels are dense and heavy—half is all you get.

The small amount of milk you use in coffee or tea needn't be counted.

Coffee and tea present no special problems for the diabetic.

Artificial sweeteners may be used (unless you are pregnant).

Obviously you won't use real syrup on your pancakes or French toast. Use only tub margarine or add a *little* dietetic syrup or jelly.

If you take insulin, always be sure to eat the same amount of carbohydrate every morning. Your dose of insulin is predicated on the food you eat. When you eat less, you may have a reaction. When you eat more, you may raise your sugar level. Always have the same kind of breakfast with the same combination of starches and proteins.

To help you plan breakfast, here are the carbohydrate values of 1 cup of some popular cereals. Not included are the sugarcoated varieties, which you must not eat. Note that Grape-Nuts are very high in carbohydrate and that the bran cereals are also high. Avoid Grape-Nuts and eat only ½ cup of bran cereal or Wheat Chex for your equivalent of two slices of bread.

Cereal (1 cup)	Grams of carbohydrate
All-Bran	44
Bran Buds	72
Cheerios	23
Cornflakes	24
40% Bran Flakes	30
Grape-Nuts	92

Cereal (1 cup)	Grams of carbohydrate
Grapenut Flakes	31
100% Bran	69
Nutrigrain	32
Puffed Rice	12.8
Puffed Wheat	8
Raisin Bran	47
Rice Krispies	24
Special K	22
Shredded Wheat (2 biscuits)	41
Total	30
Weetabix (2 biscuits)	28
Wheat Chex	52
Wheaties	24

LUNCH AND DINNER

Eat whatever you wish, but try to have a balanced meal. Avoid refined sugars and eat no more than 40 to 45 grams of carbohydrate. Include some vegetables as well as protein, which converts slowly to carbohydrate. If your weight and cholesterol are normal, you may have whatever amount of proteins and fats you are accustomed to eating. If not, see page 64.

Be sure that every meal includes the equivalent of two slices of bread; or, in other words, two units of the "big" starches found in the 15-gram list. You will need this slowly absorbed carbohydrate to carry you over until your next meal or snack. If all your carbohydrate is taken in the form of fruit or juices (10-gram list), it may throw your blood sugar into a tailspin. On the other hand, always include as well a selection from the 10-gram list to provide the blood sugar you will need in the next couple of hours.

If you don't like eating bread for lunch, you can substitute other foods. Try this, for example. It is the equivalent of two slices of bread and it's tasty: one 8-ounce container of plain yogurt, topped with a cup of strawberries or half a cup of blueberries or four inches of banana, and a little non-sugar sweetener.

Your lunch may consist of meat or fish, 2 slices of bread or a starch equivalent, one 3-percent vegetable, one 6-percent vegetable. Plus coffee, tea, or a diet drink.

For most insulin-taking diabetics, however, it's best not to eat fruit at lunch because it can raise your blood sugar too much. The long-acting insulin you've taken in the morning won't peak until about 3 P.M.

For example, perhaps you will choose for lunch:

- 3 ounces of meat (0 carbohydrate)
- Salad with lettuce and ½ cup tomatoes (6 grams carbohydrate), with French dressing (1 tablespoon or 3½ grams)
- 2 slices of bread (30 grams)

This adds up to 39½ grams of carbohydrate, right in the ballpark.

For dinner, perhaps you will eat:

- 3 to 6 ounces of chicken (0 carbohydrate)
- 1 ear of corn (30 grams)
- ½ cup of peas (6 grams)
- ½ grapefruit (10 grams)

You have a total of 46 grams of carbohydrate. Always include a 10-gram fruit at dinner.

On special occasions, it is permissible to substitute a piece of marble or pound cake for your bread allowance, if the cake weighs the same as a slice of bread.

SNACKS
Diabetics who take Regular or NPH insulin should always add two or three snacks to their three meals so

their blood sugar never sinks too low. Usually, an afternoon and an evening snack are sufficient, but if you tend to get shaky before lunch, add one in the morning. Diabetics on diet alone, oral agents, or the newer insulins without peaks (Lantus, Levemir or Apidra) do not need the snacks because they will almost never have too much insulin in their bloodstreams.

Midmorning: About 10:30 (if you have had your breakfast at 7 or 8 A.M.), those taking Regular or NPH must eat 10 grams of carbohydrate. Perhaps you'll choose 2 graham crackers, or 3 Social Teas, or a small orange, or a glass of milk.

Midafternoon: About 3 or 4 P.M., have another 10 or 15 grams of carbohydrate if you take Regular insulin before lunch.

Before bed: Eat 15 grams of carbohydrate *plus* some protein before you go to sleep. The protein will slowly convert to carbohydrate during the night, warding off early-morning insulin reactions. The only exception to this snack is if you've had a very late dinner, leaving you no time for more food.

Suggestions: 1 slice of bread and a slice of cheese; a glass of milk; half a glass of milk with crackers; one fruit and ½ slice of cheese; half a chicken or tuna sandwich; a scoop of ice cream; peanut butter and crackers.

By the way, you don't have to buy packaged snack bars for your snacks. Regular food will do the job and is far less expensive.

NOTE: the carbohydrate content of the snacks is *in addition to* your 40 to 45 grams per meal. Don't save it from your meals.

NO INSULIN, NO SNACKS!

Scheduled snacks are required for diabetics who take Regular or NPH insulin but, except for 3-percent vegetables, they are not allowed for those who are controlled by diet or oral hypoglycemic agents. What, no snack before bed? That's right.

On the other hand, if that edict is too cruel for you to live with, here's a compromise: Save a fruit or the equivalent of a slice of bread from dinner and have it before you go to bed.

FREE FOODS

Along with the 3-percent raw vegetables, these are foods you can eat as you like because they contain very little or no carbohydrate, or they are used in such small amounts as to be insignificant. For example, 1 ounce of soy sauce has only 2.7 grams of carbohydrate.

Artificial sweeteners
Bouillon
Celery salt
Cinnamon
Dietetic candy and gum (up to 5 pieces a day)
Dietetic gelatin (up to 1 cup a day)
Dietetic jams and jellies
Garlic
Herbs and spices
Horseradish
Lemon
Mayonnaise
Mint
Monosodium glutamate
Mustard
Pepper
Sour or unsweetened dill pickles
Soy sauce
Sugar-free sodas
Tartar sauce
Vinegar
Worcestershire sauce

DIET FOR DUMMIES

The diet we've outlined should be easy for almost anybody to follow, but if all else fails, remember these four simple rules:

1. No double starches. If you have bread at a meal, you can't have a potato. If you have corn, you can't have rice. If you have cereal and milk for breakfast, you must not have bread too. One starch per meal is all you're allowed.

2. No opaque soups. Don't eat soup that you can't see through (gazpacho is the exception). Stay away from such soups as pea, barley, lentil, and vegetable.

3. No apples or pineapples. Except for very small apples, they have too much carbohydrate for one sitting unless you exercise a lot, are taking enough insulin to cover it, or are only a mild diabetic.

4. No more than two fruits a day. Exception: If you are on Regular or NPH insulin, you may have another one as your 3 P.M. snack.

IF YOU NEED TO LOSE WEIGHT

It's estimated that over 190 million Americans, adults and children, are overweight, and 90 million are obese. Take yourself off the list and you'll have a good chance of losing your diabetes, cutting down on your medications, or at least not progressing further down the primrose path.

To turn this easy carbohydrate-counting diabetic diet into a weight-loss diet, all you have to do is limit the amount of proteins and fats you consume. Remember that with weight loss many adult diabetics can "lose" their disease for years, maybe forever. Others can cut down on their insulin or oral-agent requirements. Some-

times the loss of only a few pounds is enough to reduce
your insulin resistance so that your available insulin is
now adequate without outside help.

ARE YOU OVERWEIGHT?

If you are too heavy, it is imperative to shed some
pounds, especially if you are an "apple," a person who
is fattest around the middle. You can determine whether
you need to lose weight by calculating your body mass
index (BMI). A BMI of 25 or more raises your risk of
diabetes if you don't already have it, and may be what's
keeping you diabetic if you do.

Your BMI is your weight divided by your height
squared. Follow these rules: First, multiply your weight
in pounds by 705. Divide the result by your height in
inches, then divide that result by your height in inches
again. For example, if you weigh 200 pounds and are 5
feet 8 inches tall: 200 multiplied by 705 equals 141,000;
divided by 68 (inches) once, is 2,073; divided by 68
again, is a little over 30. At a body mass index of 30, you
are overweight. Try for a BMI of 25 or less.

GET OUT THE TAPE MEASURE

If you're not good at math, all you have to do is measure
yourself around the waist. A recent study has found that
waist-to-hip ratio is a good predictor of heart attack
and diabetes: A ratio (waist measurement divided by hip
measurement) below 0.85 in women or 0.9 in men is average. Anything above that increases the risk. Or, even
simpler, your waist should be no larger than 40 inches if
you're a man, and 35 inches if you're a woman.

Another study linked big bellies with a much higher

risk of type 2 diabetes, with the risk increasing along with the abdominal fat.

RULES FOR DIABETICS ON A DIET

Do not cut back on your 40 to 45 grams of carbohydrate per meal or your snacks if you take insulin. These are essential to your health. Besides, they are not nearly so fattening as fats and almost all protein foods (most of which have a high percentage of fat), a fact which continues to amaze people who have heard all their lives that bread and potatoes are what put on weight. Too many calories is what puts on weight. Fats and the majority of protein foods contain many more calories than starches.

Proteins do slow down the absorption of food and make you feel more satisfied. In fact, there's a well-known story in medical circles about the Canadian fur trapper who, back in 1826, was shot in the abdomen, allowing his digestive process to be observed by his doctor, who decided to perform an experiment. He fed the poor man a piece of bread on a string, then a piece of meat on a string, and found that the bread went down much faster than the meat.

To lose weight, eat less fat (butter, cream, margarine, oil, cream cheese, nuts, etc.) and stay away from fried foods. Limit your meat or fish portion to 3 ounces at lunch and dinner. Each 3-ounce portion of meat or fish adds 217 calories. You will now have (including your allotted carbohydrates) a 1,000-calorie diet. Remember, you must eat enough carbohydrate to provide the body's essential fuel and prevent acidosis, so *do not* lower your allotment. If you wish to lose more slowly, you may eat 3 ounces of meat or fish for lunch and 6 ounces for dinner.

You will surely be eating less than you did before, if

you pay attention to your portions. Many people eat perfectly healthy diets but their portions are totally out of control, in part because so many restaurants today serve each diner enough for two or three hearty eaters. If you can restrain yourself from eating all of it, you'll profit. You won't gain weight and you'll have enough for tomorrow. Don't be timid. Take it home in a bag.

DON'T GO OVERBOARD

But don't cut back on your calories too strenuously. Women should never eat fewer than 1,000 to 1,200 calories a day, and men at least 1,200 to 1,400 calories a day. Fewer than that and you will start losing muscle tissue instead of fat.

If you're walking around feeling famished, load up on raw 3-percent vegetables. You can eat as much as you want and they will make you feel full. The same with water. Drink 8 ounces before a meal or any other time you feel like it and you'll take the edge off your appetite.

If you take insulin, you cannot cut your usual calories without adjusting your dose. So, before you go on a diet, discuss it with your doctor. This is very important.

If you take oral agents, you probably won't require a change in dosage, but talk it over with your doctor before beginning your new regimen.

If you are on diet alone, you have no problem.

NEED HELP?

If you would like to lose weight and maybe your diabetes but can't seem to do it on your own, consult your physician about drugs that may help. There are quite a few on the market today, including some that have been around for the past thirty years, such as Tenuate Dospan and ionamin, and are still prescribed.

Others that have come along more recently, such as Meridia and Orlistat seem to be effective and safe.

Accomplia, long ago approved in England, and which may get a new name here, seems to have some special attributes that will surely make it a big seller, if they pan out to be valid. It targets the pleasure center in the brain that is linked to overeating, and acts as a cannaboid inhibitor to diminish appetite. Not only that, but it seems to increase HDL, lower triglycerides, *and* help nicotine addicts stop smoking.

It's important, of course, never to take any of these drugs without a doctor's supervision.

CAUTION: Beware of unregulated diet drugs sold in pharmacies, herbal shops, and health-food stores. They may not be safe and, in fact, could be dangerous.

SURGERY: THE LAST RESORT

Some extremely obese people have found that a drastic weight-loss treatment, gastric bypass surgery, is the only way to pare down their bodies. A last resort, surgery can vastly improve diabetes, according to a recent study at the University of Pittsburgh Medical Center. A serious procedure that decreases the size of the stomach by stapling or banding most of it shut, or bypassing most of it, it makes people feel satisfied with less food and restricts food absorption as well. Banding, done by laparoscopy through small incisions in the abdomen, seems to be the most popular procedure today. It works like a rubber band, tying off a section of the stomach, and is less risky than the major surgery required for bypassing or stapling.

Nevertheless, any way you do it, this is this is a big-deal operation and should not be undertaken lightly, but it is worth considering if absolutely nothing else has done the job. It has changed the lives of many obese diabetics, sometimes even ridding them of the disease in addition to lowering their blood pressure and cholesterol levels, and accomplishing other good things. In fact, most diabetics' sugar levels will become normal within a few days after the surgery, requiring close monitoring to adjust insulin levels. Oral agents can usually be stopped altogether.

Of course, if you gain the weight back after the surgery, you'll revert to your original situation, diabetes and all.

GET GOING!

It's easier for most people to attack sloth with an exercise program than to attack gluttony by cutting back on food. Besides, exercise is one of the best ways to lose weight as well as keep your diabetes under control, so try to add some vigorous physical activity to your life (see Chapter 4).

Remember, however, that diabetes control is always a balancing act between food intake and energy expenditure. Especially if you take insulin, you must not change your routine without consulting your physician because you may find yourself flat on the gym floor with an insulin reaction.

DON'T FOOL AROUND WITH THE DOSE

Diabetic teenage girls often skip their insulin injections because they want to lose weight, according to a study at the Hospital for Sick Children in Toronto. Typically, youngsters with diabetes gain about ten pounds when they start taking insulin. Some of them, desperately eager to be thin, decide to skimp on their prescribed dose, thereby putting themselves at risk for diabetic complications. The researchers found 86 percent of girls with eating problems showed early stages of diabetic retinopathy (eye damage) compared to 24 percent of those with normal eating habits.

The moral: whatever your age, never take it upon yourself to skip or reduce your prescribed insulin dose. The results can be disastrous.

BRITTLE DIABETICS, BEWARE

Brittle diabetics, those people on insulin whose blood sugar unpredictably shoots up and down in a flash, must be particularly vigilant about limiting the amount of carbohydrate they eat. Sometimes just 10 extra grams can triple their blood sugar, raising it to unacceptable and dangerous levels. So, if you are in this category, count your carbohydrates carefully and try to be absolutely consistent.

MEAT AND FISH

Here is what 3 ounces (about 217 calories) of meat or fish amounts to:

Lean beef:	Hamburger	1 large patty
	Sliced beef	2 slices, 4" × 4" × ¼" each
	Stew	½ cup meat
	Steak	1 small steak

Lamb:	Roast	2 slices, 3" × 3" × ½"
	Chop	2 ribs
	Stew	½ cup meat
Liver:		2 slices, 3" × 3" × ¼"
Pork:	Chop	1 large chop
	Roast	1 slice, 3" × 3" × ¼"
Veal:	Chop	1 medium chop, ½" thick
	Roast	1 slice, 3" × 3" × ¼"
Chicken:	Broiler	½ small broiler
	Roast	3 slices, 3" × 3" × ¼", or 1 leg and 1 slice
Turkey:	Roast	2 slices, 4" × 3" × ¼"
Fish:	Fresh halibut, cod, salmon, perch, bass, trout	1 slice, 3" × 3" × 1"
	Tuna	¾ cup (water packed)

For each ounce of meat, substitutions are:

1 slice American cheese
2 strips bacon
2 ounces creamed cottage
  cheese
1 medium egg

1 ounce fish
1 tablespoon peanut butter
5 shrimp, oysters, clams, or
  scallops

HOW MANY CALORIES DO YOU NEED?

To maintain their weight just where it is, most adults require 10 calories per pound, plus 3 calories per pound for minimal activity, 5 calories per pound for moderate exertion, and 10 calories per pound for strenuous exertion, every day.

In addition, pregnant women require an additional 300 calories a day and those who are breast-feeding need an extra 500 calories a day.

GET THAT CHOLESTEROL DOWN

Diabetics have a tendency to develop abnormally high levels of cholesterol and/or triglycerides, a situation that leads to heart disease and atherosclerosis (hardening of the arteries). See Chapter 10. If your test results are way up there, it would be extremely wise to make some changes in your diet by limiting your intake of fats, especially the saturated varieties. Your total cholesterol level should be under 200 mg/dl; triglycerides less than 150; and LDL, the undesirable cholesterol, below 100 and preferably in the 70s. HDL, the good cholesterol, should be at least 40 mg/dl for men and 50 mg/dl for women.

As for triglycerides, fats transported by the blood along with the cholesterol, they can be elevated by poor diabetic control, too much alcohol, and/or excessive consumption of sweets.

Diet can often reduce an abnormally high level of cholesterol at least to some degree, so we recommend that you try. It helps to remember that fat has 280 calories an ounce, or 9 per gram—twice the calories of carbohydrate or protein.

Avoid the foods that contain saturated animal fat and are hard, such as cheese or butter. Cut back on fatty meats, eggs, liver, and other organ meats. Though most liquid fats are made from vegetables and are unsaturated, some, such as coconut or palm oil, should be crossed off your list, and others, such as cottonseed oil, limited. Never use butter because it is saturated fat. Use soft tub margarine. Good choices are Benecol, Olivio, Smart Choice, and TakeControl, which have cholesterol-lowering effects. When margarine is hardened into bars, it becomes partially saturated.

Your goal should be to limit your total fat intake to 30 percent, with less than 10 percent coming from saturated fats. Ask yourself how often you eat hot dogs, sausages, fatty meats, cheese, doughnuts, cookies, cakes, pies, oily or creamy dressings, potato chips, butter, hard margarine, eggs, whole milk, and premium ice cream. If the answer is more than occasionally, you need to reform.

Never fry your food. Instead, bake, broil, poach, or steam. Cook with lemon juice, mustard, spices and herbs, garlic, onion, extracts, artificial sweeteners, vinegar, canola or corn oil. When eating out, ask for sauces and dressings on the side, and don't order fried foods.

Many people are lucky because they can eat all the high-cholesterol foods, such as meat and eggs, they want without affecting their cholesterol levels. They are born with more lipoprotein lipase, the enzyme that keeps their cholesterol under control.

If you aren't among the lucky ones and your cholesterol level is elevated, it is safe for you as a diabetic to take a cholesterol-lowering drug such as Pravachol, Lescol, Zocor, Mevacor, Crestor, Zetia, or Lipitor.

If your triglyceride levels are also way up there, you can add Lopid or perhaps Omnicor, which will lower your triglycerides as well as your LDL cholesterol. Antara, another filirate long used in Europe and now sold in the U.S., will also lower your triglycerides.

Some drugs can give you muscle aches or other unpleasant side effects, so switch around until you find one that agrees with you. And when you take any of these medications, remember that you should be monitored with periodic blood tests for possible liver or muscle damage.

FAST FOODS: SAFE FOR DIABETICS?

In today's hectic world, families no longer eat home-cooked meals every night and lunches are often taken on the run. For this reason, we should all know the carbohydrate values of the ready-to-eat food we may encounter.

Take, for example, hamburgers: A hamburger roll, top and bottom, is the equivalent of 2 slices of bread (30 grams of carbohydrate). The meat within is your protein. Do not overdo the catsup, since 1 tablespoon equals about 4½ grams of carbohydrate. Salad dressing also contains some sugar, but a small amount won't matter. Skip the French fries unless you are exercising strenuously or doing some heavy manual labor and need the extra grams of carbohydrate (15 French fries equal 30 grams). Forget the cola (except sugarless) and the milk shake. They are not for you.

As for pizza parlors, remember 1 slice of pizza equals almost 2 slices of bread, or 30 grams.

Now let's consider "fish 'n' chips." The batter counts as a bread. Fifteen French fries would be the equivalent of 2 slices of bread. Go easy on the coleslaw because it probably contains sugar.

MORE HELPFUL HINTS

• A banana is a banana, whether it is green, yellow, or purple, and contains about the same amount of carbohydrate even if it is called a plantain.

• Fructose is not for you because it is converted very quickly into glucose and raises your blood sugar accordingly. The more diabetic you are—meaning the less natural insulin you have available—the quicker the fructose changes to glucose.

• Apple, pineapple, grape, and prune juices, even unsweetened, are all no-nos because their sugars are much too rapidly absorbed into the bloodstream.

• Whole apples, too, frequently affect glucose tolerance adversely and should be avoided by most diabetics and hypoglycemics. A decent-size apple often contains 30 grams of rapidly metabolized sugar.

• For the same reason, stay away from applesauce, even if it is unsweetened. It is loaded with natural sugar.

• It won't help you a bit to toast your bread or eat it stale. It still retains its carbohydrate content and has merely lost its water content.

• Most cheeses, even processed, contain less than 5 grams of carbohydrate per serving, so you rarely have to worry about them when you are counting carbohydrates. Ricotta and cottage cheese have more carbs than the others, so don't go overboard with them.

• Common pitfalls are dried fruits—raisins, prunes, dried figs, pineapple, apricots, etc. They are *very* high in concentrated sugar.

• Go easy on nuts, too. A few won't hurt you, but a lot may send your blood sugar sky high. A pregnant woman from Hong Kong was referred to this office because she had developed diabetes. Warning her against the cashews and the lichee nuts to which she was devoted was all that was necessary. Seven cashews or six lichee nuts contain as much sugar as a fruit. As for other nuts, 30 pistachios, 22 peanuts, 10 walnuts, or 15 almonds are equal in carbohydrate to half a fruit portion. A couple of nuts won't destroy you, but if you eat more than that, count them as all or part of a fruit.

SOUP MAY BE A DISASTER

• Soups frequently are the cause of a blood-sugar disaster. One patient had a very erratic pattern, with reactions one day, high sugars the next, and decided she was a brittle diabetic. It turned out the brittleness was in the soup she was eating. She ate lunch at the same restaurant every day, always ordering the soup of the day. The thick soups—barley, lentil, pea, or minestrone vegetable soups—made her sugar soar. Because of the beans, all of these soups contain astonishing concentrations of carbohydrate, too much for one meal. The days she had plain chicken soup were the days she had insulin reactions.

The soups you can eat without worry include: chicken, onion, some tomato soups, mushroom, celery, zucchini, gazpacho, cucumber—the plain soups.

If you eat creamed soup or chowders made with flour, omit one of your two units of starch for that meal. The same applies for heavy gravies.

Borscht is made from beets that are high in sugar, so it should be crossed off your list.

Miso soup is another one to avoid—a half cup contains 38.6 grams of carbohydrate, the equivalent of more than two slices of bread.

EVEN MORE HELPFUL HINTS

• Remember, sugars and simple carbohydrates are often needed to fight off insulin reactions, but the complex carbohydrates plus protein are best if you have time and they work for you.

• When you are planning to get involved in heavy exercise or manual labor, take extra carbohydrates before you begin. Some people need 60 or 70 grams per meal to compensate for strenuous physical activity.

• On the other hand, if you are suddenly not getting your accustomed exercise—if you are in bed with a broken leg—you will require more insulin and maybe less carbohydrate. Only your blood tests will give you the answer.

• Avoid "instant" breakfasts and yogurt containing *anything*. The fruits and flavors that are added are usually sugar-laden.

• A few slices of raw onion on a hamburger or in a salad won't hurt you, but remember that 5 or 6 pearl (or larger) cooked onions in a stew equal about 8 grams of carbohydrate. Proceed with caution. The same with tomatoes—a big ripe tomato that tastes so good right out of the garden can throw your sugar way off.

MORE FOODS TO WATCH OUT FOR

There are so many sugar traps lurking around that it might be helpful to be aware of a few of the more common pitfalls. These are foods you may never have suspected of containing inordinate amounts of sugar, but could throw your glucose tolerance for a real loop.

• The most popular brand of catsup contains 29 percent sugar. A tablespoon on your hamburger can be tolerated, though.

• If you use a lot of artificial sweeteners, be aware that one package contains 1 gram of sugar, so 4 to 5 packages throughout the day will add up to a lump of sugar. A patient who drank 25 cups of coffee a day (not a good idea for anyone) added a packet of sweetener to each cup, adding up to the equivalent of five teaspoons of sugar—and wondered why his blood sugar was out of control.

• Many processed foods contain amazing amounts of hidden sugar. Learn to read labels before eating concocted foods.

• Other foods with high sugar content include All-

Bran, 100% Bran, Bran Buds, Raisin Bran, Grape-Nuts, and, of course, all sugarcoated cereals.

• Beware of "milk imitations," such as nondairy creamers, fake whipped cream, etc. Most of them contain sugar as well as a long list of chemicals. Always ask for fresh milk for your coffee.

• Be careful about the amount of juice you drink. Three ounces of orange juice, for example, gives you 10 grams of sugar. Don't drink 8 ounces because it will send you right over the top. Switch to water.

• Maybe you feel virtuous because you're drinking nonalcoholic beer instead of the real stuff, but remember that it contains plenty of carbohydrate, so take it easy.

• Never substitute "fruit drinks" for fruit juice. They are not only mostly water, which you can get almost free at home, but they are made with lots of sugar. On the other hand, cranberry juice is always diluted with water, making it a fruit drink, because it is too powerful on its own. The regular "cranberry juice cocktail" contains about 32 grams of sugar per 6 ounces. So the low-calorie version—a 6-ounce portion with only 8.5 grams of sugar—is obviously a better choice for you.

YOU ARE THE BOSS

• Always take responsibility for your own food. Even hospital dietitians have been known to serve the wrong foods to diabetics, so you must monitor your food just as you do at home, counting your carbohydrates. For example, apple juice, prune juice, and grape juice are frequently found on the hospital breakfast tray. These may not be bowls of granulated sugar nor are they chocolate cookies, but they are still not right for you because they contain too much quickly absorbed sugar

that will surely swamp you, especially when you are sick
or not exercising.

Perhaps you'll be offered 8 ounces of orange juice (almost 27 grams of quick sugar) as part of your breakfast.
It is doubtful you can handle that amount of quick sugar
at one time. Or you may be given too many starches at
once—bread, corn, potatoes, all in the same meal, for
example—which will far exceed your carbohydrate limits, especially when you are in bed and getting no exercise, and even more especially when you will probably
get fruit for dessert and perhaps a 6-percent vegetable.
At breakfast, don't eat both a roll and a bowl of cereal
with milk—that's too much carbohydrate at one time.

Don't eat foods you know are not right for you, even
if they arrive on your hospital tray. Argue every debat-
able item with your doctor and/or the dietitian. Remember you are not exempt from your usual eating pattern
just because you are in the hospital. As a matter of fact,
now is the time to watch your food more carefully than
usual because your illness may make you especially sensitive to fluctuating blood-sugar levels.

• Cottage cheese, pot cheese, cream cheese, sour
cream, and other cheeses, though they are milk products, cannot be substituted for milk or yogurt as part of
your carbohydrate allotment, but you can include them
in your diet as you wish as a protein. No restrictions unless you wish to lose weight.

• Breaded foods count toward your total carbohydrates. Omit the equivalent of 1 slice of bread (15
grams) when you eat them.

• Read labels! Some "health" foods, such as Tofutti,
contain honey or other forms of sugar and will raise
blood sugar in a hurry.

SPICING UP YOUR SALAD

• If you use just a tablespoon or two of prepared salad dressings, you can get away with most of them. Check the labels to determine their sugar content. When in doubt, make your own dressing or flavor your salad with wine vinegar or lemon, plus spices. You may add oil unless you are trying to lose weight. It contains no carbohydrate.

To help you, here are the carbohydrate values of a few prepared salad dressings.

Salad dressing (1 tablespoon)	Grams of carbohydrate
Caesar	1.0
French	3.5
Vinaigrette	1.4
Italian	0.7
Red wine vinegar, oil	4.0
Mayonnaise	3.5
Russian	4.5

Though most salad dressings do not contain much carbohydrate, they are usually laden with calories, a fact to keep in mind if you are overweight. Most low-calorie dressings contain fewer (some far fewer) than 3 grams of carbohydrate per tablespoon, but others have more. Read the labels.

Beware of coleslaw—it may contain a lot of mayonnaise and sugar.

TIMING YOUR FOOD

If you take insulin, *when* you eat is just as important as *what* you eat. *All* diabetics should space out their carbohydrate intake throughout the day so that there won't be high peaks and low valleys in blood-sugar levels. But when you're on insulin, you must also worry about reactions. It's important that you eat at specified times because, like a time bomb, the hormone acts at fixed hours of the day. If you don't have food in anticipation of these periods of high insulin action, you will have reactions. You have more flexibility if your regime calls for Regular or one of the newer fast-acting insulins just before meals. This is a big help to one patient who is an actor and never knows when he'll get a chance to eat a meal.

Never skip a meal or a planned snack. Do not delay your meals. If you are going to a party and know dinner will be served later than your usual mealtime, eat 30 grams of your carbohydrate at your usual time. Then, when you get to the dinner party, skip those 30 grams of carbohydrate (rolls, potatoes, pilaf, etc.) and eat the main course, salad, vegetables, and fruit for dessert. Do not take a chance that you may last until your hostess or the restaurant serves you. Plan ahead or you'll spoil the whole affair for everyone.

With some of the new fast-acting insulins, however, strict adherence to a rigid eating schedule is not anywhere near as important as it is with Regular or NPH. Lantus or Levemir, supplemented with Humalog, Novo-Log, or Apridra taken before meals, won't give you major peaks of insulin that must be covered by food, and so are not likely to cause insulin reactions if you don't eat on time. The supplemental doses of fast-acting insulin are taken just before or after your meals, which means that you can safely put lunch off for an hour or two, or even skip a meal, although we don't recommend that.

The same is true with the oral drugs Prandin and Starlix, because they too are taken with meals and offer the same kind of flexibility.

HOW TO BE A HAPPY DINER

Once you know the general rules of diet for a diabetic, then you can apply your common sense when you're eating out. For example, you go to a Chinese restaurant and start with an egg roll. The coating on the egg roll is roughly equivalent to a slice of bread (15 grams of carbohydrate). Now eat a simple main dish, perhaps fish or meat with vegetables, and you can still have the equivalent of another slice of bread. That means a ½ cup of rice or noodles. The carbohydrate value of Chinese soups is negligible if you avoid those containing sugar, such as sweet and sour soup. If you have wonton soup, count three wontons as one bread. Don't eat the duck sauce. Avoid sweet sauces. But have a fortune cookie for good luck.

Using the same common sense, you can eat without fear in any restaurant. When you're out for an Italian dinner, consider a small order of spaghetti to be roughly equal to 2 slices of bread and a fruit. Skip the bread and the bread sticks (two bread sticks equal one bread). Eat the main course and a salad. Italian soups can be a problem because they usually have too much carbohydrate for you. If you skip your two breads and a fruit, you can have two cups of cooked pasta with olive oil and garlic, or pesto, clams, or primavera. But not tomato sauce, which is too high in quickly absorbed sugar. Forget dessert.

At a Middle Eastern restaurant, a regular-size pita counts as two breads. Tabbouleh is a starch just like rice. Shish kebab is no problem. Chickpeas, hummus, fava beans, and spinach pies are all heavy starch. Go easy.

Don't order sukiyaki in a Japanese restaurant because it includes questionable amounts of sugar and/or sweet wine. Count the batter coating as a bread exchange when eating tempura. Stay with the simple dishes such as mizutaki—beef or chicken chunks cooked in broth. And remember what we said about miso soup—skip it.

TO FAST OR NOT TO FAST

Religious fast days such as Yom Kippur can complicate the lives of diabetics who take insulin. If you are controlled by diet alone, fasting is no problem. If you take oral drugs, it is no problem either, but it might be best to skip your pill in the morning and take it before the evening meal that breaks the fast.

For insulin users, fasting is much trickier, and in most cases you would be wise not to try it. Surely your need for food when you are diabetic will not alter the effectiveness of your prayers. It might be better to bend the traditional rules than to encounter a medical emergency.

If fasting is very important to you, however, it can be done. Suppose you normally take 10 Regular and 30 units of Intermediate insulin in the morning. If today is a fast day, take no insulin in the morning, have no breakfast or lunch. Suppose the day goes by and you remain asymptomatic. Check your blood before dinner. If you find you have high sugar (almost a sure bet), do *not* take your usual morning dose. Take more Regular than usual (to compensate for the higher-than-normal sugar) and less Intermediate (because you don't want it to last through the next day). For example: 20 Regular and 20 Intermediate.

But suppose, without insulin, breakfast, and lunch, you begin having symptoms of high sugar and acidosis—frequent urination, thirst, etc. *Do not wait* for dinner. Break the fast *immediately*. Start eating and take your insulin, again increasing your Regular to take care of the high sugar and cutting back on your Intermediate insulin.

If you take Lantus or Levemir at bedtime the night before you fast, it would probably be wise to take only half your usual dose because you will have a lot of insulin on board when you eat nothing the next day.

Do not do any of the above without consulting your own doctor!

COMMENTS ON "CHEATING"

There are very few perfect people in this world, and diabetics are no more likely to be among them than anyone else. It is a rare diabetic who doesn't cheat on his prescribed diet once in a while. This is not the end of the world and you shouldn't feel too guilty about it. But it is *not* a good idea to fall off your diet regularly because, if you do, your control will automatically be poor and you will be subject to all the ills and complications that befall poorly controlled diabetics.

For insulin-taking people who cheat occasionally, it is possible to compensate for a binge by taking a blood test after the event and taking a few extra units of fast-acting Regular insulin if you see very high sugar.

The best way to cheat, however, is to do your forbidden eating before you set off on a program of strenuous exercise, when you may need extra carbohydrates anyway. For example, if you are going to the movies, don't overindulge at dinner. But if your plans include a lot of vigorous dancing, you can probably plan on burning off the excess carbohydrate before the night is out.

HIGH FIBER: GOOD FOR YOU?

According to research, increased fiber in your diet can improve your glucose tolerance slightly. Some fiber foods, such as pectin, guar, and oat bran, are water-soluble. They delay absorption of carbohydrates by trapping them within themselves and releasing them slowly. Because of the delay, less sugar enters the bloodstream immediately after a meal, avoiding an overload. This kind of fiber also seems to lower the level of cholesterol in the blood.

Other fibers, such as cellulose, lignin, and wheat bran, are not water-soluble. They pass through the digestive system quickly, taking other foods along with them, giving the intestines less opportunity to absorb carbohydrates. These also soften the stool and add bulk to it.

The canes, roots, and tubers that, before we became so civilized, once constituted the major part of mankind's daily food have been replaced by a diet high in animal proteins and fats as well as grain cereals that have lost most of their fiber content in the milling process. The typical Western diet includes only about 4 grams of crude fiber a day. In some less-developed countries it makes up 30 grams of the daily diet, and is associated with lower incidences of diabetes, diverticulitis, appendicitis, hemorrhoids, and cancer of the colon. On the other hand, except for lignin found in strawberries and pears, it increases flatulence (gas).

Fiber is indigestible, unabsorbable plant material and is not found in meat or fish. It leaves the digestive system in much the same form it went in and has virtually no caloric value. Nevertheless, it plays a number of vital roles in the digestive process. It is found chiefly in whole grains, nuts and beans, fruits, and vegetables, especially those with edible skins and seeds. It does not matter whether these foods are eaten raw, cooked, frozen, or canned.

Should you, a diabetic, eat a high-fiber diet? More fiber, especially grains, certainly will not hurt you and may well give you an extra little edge. It won't cure your diabetes, but it could tip the scales in your favor. In fact, a large and respected Harvard study of 65,000 healthy women showed that those who ate lots of fiber-rich whole grains—especially in breakfast cereals—had a 28 percent lower risk of developing type 2 diabetes. And a study at the University of Texas Southwestern Medical Center at Dallas, reported in 2000, found that a diet high in fiber, especially the soluble variety, leads to improved glycemic control and lower cholesterol and triglyceride levels in type 2 diabetics.

That's fine but you can easily lose control of your blood sugar by increasing your dietary fiber too much, because it almost always contains major amounts of carbohydrate. Five grams of fiber is roughly equivalent to 1 gram of carbohydrate. So tread carefully and don't go overboard. Be sure to include these foods in your carbohydrate allotment for the day.

If you are on diet alone or oral agents, you may find that your available insulin is more effective with more fiber. And if you take insulin you may require a little less of the medication. Fiber isn't, however, a cure-all; there is a limit to the amount of it you can eat safely, because most fiber foods are high-starch compounds that take time to be broken down but nonetheless are absorbed as carbohydrate at some time during their metabolism. Among the fiber foods, peas and baked beans have been found to raise blood sugar more than the others.

Important: Remember to include the fiber foods in your 40 to 45 grams of carbohydrate per meal. Dried beans and bran cereals, for example, tend to be high-carbohydrate foods. Two tablespoons of bran or wheat germ equal about 15 grams of carbohydrate, and you must account for it in your total allotment. Keep in mind that two-thirds of a cup of beans is the equivalent of 2 slices of bread or 30 grams of carbohydrate. Eat a big bowl of beans and you are in trouble, so pay attention to your portions.

FOODS WITH FIBER

To get more fiber into your diet, you should eat:

• Whole-grain breads and cereals, especially whole bran or bran-containing foods. To make sure you're getting whole grains, check the labels. Don't be fooled by the color that's often added for cosmetic purposes or the name that can be misleading, but choose a product that lists the grains first in the list of ingredients and contains at least 2 grams of fiber, and preferably 3 grams, per serving. "Fiber breads" may be added to the list. Check the carbohydrate content of each slice so you can be sure to eat a sufficient number of grams.

• Nuts and seeds. Remember, however, their high carbohydrate content.

• Vegetables from the 3 percent variety: broccoli, cabbage, cauliflower, green peppers, cucumbers. Or the 6 percent variety: brussels sprouts, corn, peas, artichokes, red peppers, beans, and carrots, which you must account for.

• Fruits such as strawberries, blueberries, bananas, mangoes, peaches, grapefruit, and pears.

• Leguminous dried beans—butter, haricot, kidney, soy, lentils, black-eyed, or chickpeas, etc. Be careful, however. Beans are high in carbohydrates.

Caution: Sometimes the absorption of some important trace minerals, such as calcium, zinc, iron, and magnesium, is inhibited when you consume too much fiber. Their absorption, along with that of glucose, may be decreased. So don't go overboard. Eat well-balanced meals that happen to include sufficient fiber.

Some people prefer to get their extra fiber by sprinkling bran into their food. Fruits and vegetables are a much more nutritious alternative, and it is best to get your fiber the natural way, by eating properly. Remember, too, that two flat tablespoons of bran is the equivalent of a slice of bread. Surprisingly, a serving of avocado contains considerable fiber, about 12 grams.

If you are not accustomed to much fiber in your diet, work up to a higher amount gradually. If you notice too much gas or bloating, cut back until you have adjusted. Your body probably will become accustomed to it in a few weeks.

Don't eat your fiber between meals, or it won't have food to act upon. Eat it with your other food.

VITAMINS AND OTHER SUPPLEMENTS

This is an age of megavitamins, and controversy continues over the need for vitamins and minerals in addition to a balanced diet. Though most medical experts do not think people who eat a wide variety of nourishing foods require supplements unless they are deficient in them, and except for a multivitamin for people who are elderly, pregnant, vegetarian, or on a low-calorie diet, there is some thought that a few supplements may be helpful to diabetics. Let's go down the list.

Vitamin B$_1$: This is a vitamin that I recommend to my patients with diabetic neuropathy (pain or burning) and about 80 percent of them show some improvement or even complete relief when they take it regularly in daily 100 mg doses. It is especially helpful for neuropathy of the feet. Sometimes injections of vitamin B_{12} also help.

Vitamin B_6: Because this is thought to increase glucose tolerance in pregnant women, a supplement of 25 mgs a day is recommended during pregnancy.

Vitamin C: Some doctors recommend C supplements because they believe it strengthens the capillary walls of the eyes and prevents diabetic eye changes.

Vitamin D, which comes from sunlight and milk, is thought to improve your ability to rid yourself of glucose and blood fats, metabolize calcium, and keep your blood pressure under control. Be sure to get enough of it. Ten minutes a day in the sun will probably give you an ample supply but just to be sure, take a daily multi-vitamin supplement that includes 400 I.U. of this important vitamin.

Vitamin E: Once called the miracle vitamin because it is a powerful antioxidant, Vitamin E was thought to protect against all manner of problems, from cancer to heart disease. Some of its benefits have not been substantiated and today, instead of the very high doses formerly recommended, we think 100 or 200 I.U. a day is plenty.

Chromium picolinate has become one of the hot dietary supplements, especially for diabetics. Among the wonders attributed to this natural trace mineral are that it lowers blood sugar, reduces body fat, controls appetite, and reduces cholesterol. However, there is still little solid scientific evidence to support any of these claims, except for the few people who are chromium deficient.

Having said all that, it remains a possibility that chromium may give your insulin supply a boost—but only *if* you have too little of it. It probably won't hurt you in daily doses of 50 to 200 micrograms from foods such as fruits and vegetables (most Americans consume about 30 micro-grams a day) and/or supplements. Talk to your doctor before deciding to take it.

Selenium is another nutrient that's moving quickly off the shelves today because of its apparent ability to raise blood levels of HDL, the desirable cholesterol, which helps protect against heart disease. However, while the promise of benefit from a daily supplement is strong, it has not yet been proved and most people get plenty of selenium from their food. Major sources include egg yolks, poultry, seafood, whole grains, and foods grown in selenium-rich soil. But because diabetics have blood vessels that can use all the help they can get, it's a good idea to take a daily supplement of 50 to 100 micrograms—if, of course, your own doctor approves.

Calcium supplements are recommended for anyone who does not drink much milk, eat a lot of milk products, or get regular exercise. It's good for your bones and your blood pressure. Be sure to consume at least 1,000 mg of calcium a day; 1,500 if you are a postmenopausal woman who does not take estrogen replacement.

Magnesium is in short supply in poorly controlled diabetics and those with severe retinopathy, although it is not yet known whether adding magnesium salts to your diet will prevent eye changes. But a recent study of 85,000 nurses suggests that people with the highest levels of magnesium in their diets have the lowest risk of getting diabetes. Your doctor can check the magnesium level in your blood and, if it is low, may suggest that you take it as a supplement. Natural sources include whole grains, fruits, vegetables, cereals, nuts, beans.

Zinc is required for normal growth and development, and some research has shown that, given orally in 200 mg doses, it helps heal diabetic ulcers. It is found naturally in green leafy vegetables, fruits, whole-grain breads, and meat. Don't overdose yourself—too much zinc will cause nausea.

DHEA, a hormone secreted by the adrenal glands and converted into small amounts of testosterone and estrogen, is claimed to combat everything from aging to obesity to AIDS. Some research suggests that it may improve insulin sensitivity but we urge you not to take it until controlled human studies are conducted and more is known about its long-term safety. As a "dietary supplement" like chromium picolinate and melatonin, it does not require FDA approval, which means its safety and effectiveness have not been scientifically evaluated and nobody knows if it is safe or what the proper dose should be.

Melatonin sold in health-food stores is a synthetic version of a human hormone and may help you sleep or overcome jet lag, but probably does little else. We recommend that you stay away from it because serious questions remain regarding proper dosage, interactions with other drugs, and long-term side effects.

Alpha-lipoic acid, otherwise known as oil of primrose, appears to improve insulin sensitivity in type 2 diabetics and relieve the discomforts of peripheral neuropathy because of its antioxidant and anti-inflammatory effects. If you are going to try it, 500 mgs three times a day should be a safe dose.

NOTE: There is no difference, except in the price, between natural and synthetic vitamins.

SPECIAL FOODS: GOOD FOR YOU?

It's not easy to keep up with the hundreds of foods and herbs that are supposed to be good for diabetics, and it's even more difficult to know whether the claims made for them have any validity whatsoever. Many have shown some promise for diabetes, but the scientific evidence for their safety and efficacy is too uncertain for experts to make recommendations about most of them.

Among the current favorites are those listed here. It is doubtful that any of them will hurt you, unless you overdo them, and some may even do you some good. Remember that a few may have an unfortunate interaction with prescription diabetes drugs, perhaps making your blood sugar levels drop too far, so don't take anything new without checking with your doctor.

Cinnamon can lower blood sugar, triglyceride and cholesterol levels, as well as improve insulin sensitivity, according to a scientist at the Human Nutrition Research Center of the U.S. Department of Agriculture. One teaspoon a day is said to be all it takes to do the job. In addition, a Pakistani team tested cinnamon capsules against placebo capsules and found that the spice made a definite difference in the reduction of blood glucose. In 2006, German researchers published new data that also supported cinnamon use for diabetics. If these findings are confirmed by wider studies, cinnamon has a great future.

Soy supplements may help prevent common diabetes complications such as kidney and heart disease, according to findings at the University of Illinois. A group of older men with diabetes-related kidney disease was divided into two smaller groups, one given soy protein powder, the other a different protein powder, mixed into foods. Those getting the soy had a 10 percent reduction in protein found in their urine.

Alcohol consumption, light to moderate, may actually be good for you. It's associated with a reduced death rate due to coronary heart disease in type 2 diabetics who are at higher than normal risk of dying because of cardiovascular events, report researchers from the University of Wisconsin. On the downside, alcohol may induce and mask potentially severe hypoglycemia and may worsen diabetic neuropathy.

Salacia oblonga is an herb used in traditional medicines in India and Sri Lanka. According to researchers at Ohio State University, it works similarly to such anti-diabetic oral medications as Precose and Glyset by binding to enzymes in the intestine that break down carbohydrates into glucose. This causes less glucose to be absorbed, thereby lowering blood sugar. Testing continues.

Cherries, sweet or tart, contain chemicals that boost insulin, at least in mice whose insulin-producing beta cells nearly doubled when exposed to anthocyanins, which, by the way, can also be found in red grapes, strawberries, blueberries, and other foods.

Black or green tea is good for diabetes, according to another study done on rodents, and it is being tested on people. It seems to have a blood-sugar-lowering effect and to inhibit diabetic cataracts. To get the same dose of tea given to the rats, a 143-pound person would have to drink four and a half 8-ounce cups of tea a day.

Walnuts incorporated into a healthy diet may help type 2 diabetics improve their cholesterol levels and reduce their risk of heart disease, according to a recent study. Walnuts contain an omega-3 fatty acid called alpha-linolenic acid or ALA. After a six-month diet of healthy foods supplemented by 8 to 10 walnuts a day, compared to similiar diets minus the walnuts, the walnut eaters showed a bigger increase in HDL cholesterol as well as a larger reduction in LDL levels.

Peanut butter and nuts: A Harvard study reported in 2002 showed that women who regularly ate peanut butter and nuts had a reduced risk of type 2 diabetes. And the more they ate, the lower their risk was. The nuts included almonds, hazelnuts, pecans, pistachios, walnuts, and peanuts. Just remember that nuts contain plenty of carbohydrates, so if you are already diabetic, eat only a few. One tablespoon of butter contains 3 grams of carbohydrate, and of all the nuts, cashews have the most.

Ginseng can interact with many drugs, including oral antidiabetic medications, and cause severe side effects. Diabetics should not take it.

NOTE: Confirmation of these findings as well as the rest of the claims in this section is still to come.

SWEETENERS: BLESSING OR DANGER?

Artificial sweeteners make life a little bit sweeter for people who can't eat sugar, and, from what we know now, there is no reason not to use them, at least in small amounts. A few years ago, experiments with rats showed an increased incidence of bladder cancer among second-generation rats fed the equivalent of 800 diet sodas sweetened with saccharin. Saccharin was promptly removed from many homes and hospitals as a result. However, subsequent research on people has failed to show any correlation between the sweetener and cancer, and saccharin (cyclamate) is now available in many brands, including Sweet'n Low, Sweet Magic, and Sugar Twin, and is considered safe.

As are the other artificial sweeteners on the market today, such as aspartame (Nutrasweet and Equal), D-tagatose (Sugaree), acesulfame potassium (Sunett), and the new guy on the block, sucralose (Splenda), which may be used in cooking. Another sweetener called Stevia, an herbal ingredient used for centuries in South America and for a few decades in Japan, is sold as a dietary supplement in health-food stores, but it has not been scientifically tested and is not FDA-approved.

All of them are good choices for diabetics, although you should remember that the sweeteners all contain approximately 1 gram of sugar per packet. So if you consume five packets of sweetener in a day, you're eating the equivalent of a lump of sugar.

For diabetics, artificial sweeteners are a much better choice than sugar and keep you from feeling like a second-class citizen. Children, especially, need to feel they are not being totally deprived of the goodies their friends consume so freely.

THE LURE OF "DIETETIC" FOODS

Just because a packaged food (usually very expensive) is labeled "dietetic," it does not mean it is good for diabetics. Although no refined sugar has been included, it may still contain much more carbohydrate than you can handle. Take, for example, dietetic apple pie. Though it may be sweetened artificially, it still has a crust and plenty of apples, and you can exceed your limit without added sugar. On the other hand, you may be able to get away with a piece of dietetic blueberry pie occasionally because it contains a lower sugar content than apple pie, and the natural sugar is not as quickly absorbed. Count the crust as two slices of bread or 30 grams of carbohydrate, and substitute the blueberries for your fruit at dinner. Guide yourself by your blood tests.

Though such items as water-packed canned fruits, dietetic jellies, and gelatin desserts can perk up your menu, many modified foods still contain too much sugar, honey, or syrup for you (though perhaps in smaller amounts than the usual recipe) as well as carbohydrates in other forms.

In general, foods called "noncaloric" or those containing only a few (under 10) calories per serving are safe, eaten in limited amounts. For example, you can safely eat small amounts of dietetic jam or candy. But stay away from dietetic cookies, cakes, chocolates, sherbets, breads, and custards, as well as liquid nondairy creamers, dietetic dinners, and diet bars. Unless you are a chemist, the listed ingredients of most processed dietetic foods are impossible to interpret correctly.

FAKED OUT BY FRUCTOSE

Once proclaimed to be the answer to a diabetic's dream of a "good" sugar, fructose has not lived up to expectations. Though this kind of sugar does not require insulin for its metabolism, it converts to glucose in the body and can raise blood-sugar levels just like any of its sugary relatives. The more deficient in insulin you are, the quicker the conversion.

Sorbitol, mannitol, ducitol, and xylitol, all sugar alcohols, are also converted to glucose, but more slowly. You may be able to handle these in tiny amounts, though some people respond to them with cramps and diarrhea.

Avoid carob, a sweetener that tastes like chocolate— it is 75 percent sugar.

SUGAR IS SUGAR

Sugar is sugar, no matter what its taste or physical form and regardless of whether it's called brown sugar, corn syrup, fruit sugar, honey, or maple syrup. And none of them is any better or worse for you or anybody else than plain white table sugar. All of these sweeteners are virtually indistinguishable and they supply nothing but empty calories. Honey and syrups are more concentrated than granulated sugar, so they pack more calories per teaspoon.

Sugar comes in many disguises. Beware of any ingredients that end in "-ose" or "-tol." These are usually just plain sugar. For example: dextrose, lactose, sorbitol. Sometimes labels list several varieties of sugar with different names, such as: dextrose, fructose, glucose, sucrose, sorbitol, mannitol, lactose, disaccharide, corn syrup, corn sugar, corn syrup solids, honey, molasses, maltose. Watch out for all of them! Add a few together in one food and you come up with a high percentage of sugar, more than you can cope with.

Legislation requires that the ingredients of most foods be listed on the label, and also the amounts in grams of carbohydrates, proteins, and fats, according to serving size. Use this information to plan your 40 to 45 grams of carbohydrate per meal.

NO SMOKING ALLOWED!

We all know by now that smoking is hazardous to everyone's health. For diabetics, who already have a tendency toward vascular disease, smoking is even more dangerous. Smoking affects the coronary blood vessels as well as the smaller vessels in the legs and feet, constricting them, reducing circulation, and affecting the ability of any damaged tissues to heal. In addition, diabetics, especially if they are not in good control, have less oxygen in their tissues than other people. Smoking raises the blood level of carbon monoxide, thus adding to that oxygen deficit. Smoking is also known to increase a tendency toward retinopathy.

If you are a smoker, do yourself an enormous favor and quit.

MARIJUANA AND OTHER DRUGS

Though there are conflicting reports about the effects of marijuana on mind and body, it is certain that this drug is not a good idea for you. For one thing, it can mask insulin reactions so you may not recognize that you need immediate food. For another thing, it could distort your sense of time so that you may not eat on schedule. And it may set off the "munchies," a craving for sweets that has obvious drawbacks. It may also lower blood pressure in the eyes, a possible prelude to bleeding if you have diabetic retinopathy.

Amphetamines (uppers) are stimulants that can raise or lower your blood sugar unexpectedly. Narcotics (heroin and cocaine) can affect the blood sugar by altering absorption of sugar. So, for these reasons, as well as many others, don't try to get your kicks from drugs.

STAY AWAY FROM GINSENG

Ginseng, a root long popular in Asia and here as well today, is said to cure many ills, but don't try it if you are diabetic. Ginseng may lower blood sugar, cause ulcers, and enlarge male breasts, and may well be damaging for anyone. And if you take ginseng in addition to diabetes pills, the ginseng can lower your blood sugar to the point where it can cause a strong hypoglycemic reaction. Diabetics should not take it.

ALCOHOL—WHAT DOES IT DO TO YOU?

Being a diabetic doesn't mean you must give up all your bad habits. You don't have to go on the wagon and become a teetotaler. On the other hand, you must be a "sensible" drinker. A drink or two a day won't hurt you, if you are in good control and remember a few facts. Actually, alcohol in moderation seems to boost blood levels of high-density lipoproteins (the "good" cholesterol), decrease chances of heart attacks, and inhibit potentially dangerous blood clots. Besides, some studies show that it may increase the body's response to insulin and promote lower blood-sugar levels, sometimes for more than 8 hours after drinking.

Stick to moderate drinking—one drink a day for women, two for men. That translates into 12 ounces of beer (preferably light), 5 ounces of wine, or 1.5 ounces of 80 percent proof distilled spirits, per serving. Imbibe too much and who knows what will happen, surely nothing good.

Alcohol has no food value and contains no nutrients, though it does add calories to your daily diet. An ounce of whiskey, for example, contains about 85 calories. *Sweet* alcoholic drinks, however, do contain some sugar.

Here are some guidelines to follow:

• Never drink on an empty stomach. Alcohol blocks the process called gluconeogenesis, the formation of glucose from protein and its release from the liver when your blood sugar is too low. Without food, you risk having a severe hypoglycemic reaction if you are on insulin. When you drink before meals, eat some hors d'oeuvres, but be sure to count them as part of your meal's allotment of carbohydrate.

• Never have more than a moderate amount of

alcohol a day, even with food. You may not be able to recognize an insulin reaction or distinguish it from intoxication. Nor may the police, if you are pulled over for erratic driving. Remember that low blood sugar and intoxication can be—and are—often confused.

• Don't change your insulin dose or diet to allow for your alcoholic drinks.

• Watch out for the "antabuse effect" if you take Diabinese, an oral hypoglycemic agent that is rarely used today. Alcohol will sometimes cause surface blood vessels to dilate, producing marked facial flushing, plus a choking sensation and maybe a headache.

• Sweet drinks do contain carbohydrate. So do the hors d'oeuvres that usually accompany drinking. Avoid sweet wines, stout, cider, ginger beer, port, liqueurs, and cordials. Don't drink sweet mixers such as tonic unless they are sugar-free, and remember that the orange juice in a screwdriver, for example, counts toward your total allotment of quick carbohydrate for that meal. So does Bloody Mary mix (mostly tomato juice).

• A drink before dinner or a glass or two of dry wine with dinner is considered permissible for most diabetics and, in fact, may even be beneficial. The acceptable list includes: Scotch, rye, whiskey, bourbon, tequila, brandy, rum, gin, sake, vodka, and light dry wine.

• To slip an occasional beer or ale into your life, omit one slice of bread or a fruit at dinner to make up for it. There are about 10 grams of carbohydrate in 8 ounces of regular beer. Some of the "light" beers contain only about 3 grams in 8 ounces. Near-beer is about the same, but some alcohol-free beers and ales have higher sugar contents, up to 7 grams in 8 ounces, so check them out before you drink them and don't forget to add them to your daily total.

AMOUNTS OF CARBOHYDRATE, ALCOHOL, AND CALORIES IN ALCOHOLIC DRINKS

Alcoholic Drinks	Amount	Total Grams	Grams of Carbohydrate	Grams of Alcohol	Calories (Approx.)
Whiskey—Bourbon, Irish, Rye, and Scotch	1 brandy glass (1 oz.)	30	none	10½–13	75–85
Brandy, Gin, Vodka, Sake, Tequila, and Rum	1 brandy glass (1 oz.)	30	none	10½–13	75–90
Liqueurs and Cordials	1 cordial glass (⅔ oz.)	20	4–10	4–7	50–80
Malt liquors—ale, beer, porter, and stout	1 glass (8 oz.)	240	7–14	7–14	80–150
WINES					
Sweet, domestic	1 wine glass (3½ oz.)	100	8–14	13–15	140–165
Sweet, imported	1 wine glass (3½ oz.)	100	3–20	1½–18	110–175
*Dry, domestic	1 wine glass (3½ oz.)	100	½–4	10–11	75–90
*Dry, imported	1 wine glass (3½ oz.)	100	½–3	8–14	60–110
CIDER					
Sweet	1 glass (8 oz.)	240	25	trace	100
Hard (fermented)	1 wine glass (3½ oz.)	100	1	5	40

*Examples of dry wine include Bordeaux, claret, graves, dry sauterne, burgundy, Chablis, dry champagne, Rhine wine, and Moselle.

• Don't get stressed out if your hostess serves food cooked with wine. The carbohydrate addition is negligible and most of the alcohol is lost in the cooking. If you take Diabinese and you suffer from the "antabuse effect," however, then you must be more careful. Ask questions before you eat.

CAN DIABETICS BE VEGETARIANS?

Vegetarian diets have become popular in America, among diabetics as well as the rest of the population. Type 1 diabetics who become vegetarians may need less insulin. Type 2s may lose weight on these diets and so improve their blood-glucose control. Will they work for you? They can, *if* you consult a dietitian for advice before you begin and are vigilant about your blood-sugar levels. You must eat a diet balanced in carbohydrates, fats, and proteins, and this is not a simple matter if you don't eat meat or fish.

It is recommended that you do not follow a strict vegetarian diet, eliminating all animal foods and eating only plants. To get the needed supply of protein, strict vegetarians consume combinations of vegetables and grains that will far exceed the levels of carbohydrate that are safe for you. Besides, this diet puts you in danger of deficiencies in important vitamins and minerals.

If your diet allows fish, eggs, and/or dairy products, being a vegetarian is not quite as tricky, though tricky it remains. The protein plant foods used to supplement fish and dairy foods are very high in carbohydrate. For example, it takes only ⅛ cup of cooked lentil, mung, pinto, red beans, or chick peas, or ¼ cup of soy beans, to equal about 15 grams of carbohydrate.

You must take care not to consume too many grams

of carbohydrate at any one time, especially not too many of the quickly absorbed variety. The usual large amounts of carbohydrate in a vegetarian diet can easily cause problems with your blood-sugar level, though the increased fiber may give you a little more leeway.

LOW-SALT DIETS

If your doctor has told you to lower your salt intake, then you must avoid every food high in salt even if it is otherwise permissible. Dry cereals, for example, tend to be high in salt as are processed meats, canned vegetables, and soups. Look for the low-salt or salt-free varieties.

LOW-POTASSIUM DIETS

Certain fruits, such as figs, pineapples, apples, raisins, and prunes, that are recommended for kidney disease are not recommended for you if you are trying to maintain a low potassium intake because their sugar is too readily absorbed. Stay with the fruits that have low potassium *and* are permissible for you, such as cranberry juice, grapefruit, grapes, peaches, berries, tangerines, pears, plums, watermelon, nectarines.

THE QUICKIE DIETS

We would all like to lose weight fast, not just a pound or two a week as the more sensible weight-loss diets suggest. Are quick diets safe for diabetics?

Keep in mind that all diets work if you consume fewer calories than you use, whether you eat a lot of fat, or vegetables, or nothing but grapefruit and lettuce. But if you are a diabetic, you should have a healthy, balanced food plan or you can get into serious trouble.

Mild diabetics on low doses of oral agents or diet alone can probably get away with the Atkins Diet, the South Beach Diet, and other quickies that feature high protein and low carbohydrate if they stay on them for only a limited amount of time, if their health is good, and if they are under medical supervision and have their doctor's approval. Some diabetics may even lose their dependency on oral drugs if they lose enough weight through one of these plans.

But for other diabetics, the fad diets can be dangerous because they are designed to burn fat and produce a state of ketosis or acidosis, exactly what diabetics don't need. Acidosis inhibits your response to insulin and can put you in the hospital.

High-protein diets are risky, too, for people with the kidney problems that are common among diabetics. A high-protein diet can make you feel satisfied longer because it takes more time for the food to make its way through your digestive system, as demonstrated by the aforementioned unfortunate Canadian trapper.

Although with high-fat, high-protein diets, carbohydrates are cut way back, you still get fewer calories than you would normally eat and so you shed pounds. But you are missing important nutrients and the carbohydrates needed to provide your body with energy. And although these gimmick diets may not be harmful for a short period of time, they are not sustainable. Nor are they healthy as a long-term lifestyle, especially for diabetics.

If you're a diabetic, you should never go entirely without starches, which the Atkins and South Beach diets prescribe for their first few weeks, because you need a balanced amount of carbohydrates. If you eat too little, cut back too much on the carbs, and do not compensate by adjusting your insulin or oral agents, you may find yourself inundated with unexpected insulin reactions.

Do not try this kind of diet on your own. Better yet, don't try it at all.

CARBOHYDRATE VALUES OF POPULAR FOODS

Food	Amount	Carbohydrate Content (Grams)
Almonds	½ cup, shelled	14
Apple	1 medium, raw	20
Artichoke, boiled	1 medium	33.5
Artichoke hearts	5–6 hearts, 3 oz.	22
Anchovies	1 oz.	0.1
Avocado	½ fruit	6.4 to 10.8
Bacon	2 slices	0.2
Baked beans	½ cup	20–30
Bamboo shoots	½ lb., raw	3.4
Banana	1 small	21
Bean sprouts	½ cup, raw	3
Beans, black	4 oz., dry	69
Beans, green or wax, fresh, boiled	½ cup	3.5
Beans, Italian	½ cup	5
Beans, lima, boiled	½ cup	17–21
Beans, pinto	½ cup, dry	61
Beans, lentil	½ cup, dry	58
Beans, garbanzo (chickpeas)	½ cup, dry	61
Beef pie, frozen	8 oz.	40
Beef, consommé or broth	1 cup	2.7
Beets, cooked	½ cup	7.4
Bread crumbs	1 tbsp.	4.7
Buckwheat groats	1 oz.	21
Cashew nuts	½ cup	20
Catsup	1 tbsp.	4.9

Food	Amount	Carbohydrate Content (Grams)
Cheesecake	⅙ of 8" cake	38.8
Chestnuts, fresh, shelled	3 large	10
Chicken pie	8 oz.	50
Chili sauce	1 tbsp.	4.6
Coconut, fresh	½ cup, grated	3.8
Coconut, dried, sweetened	½ cup	23
Cornstarch	1 tbsp.	7
Cracker crumbs, graham	1 cup	76.6
Curry powder	1 tbsp.	4.9
Dates	5	40.5
Eggnog	½ cup	17
Fig, fresh	1, small	7.6
Flour	1 oz.	21
Frankfurter	1	0.7
Gefilte fish, canned	1 piece, 4 oz.	4.2
Lasagne, canned, frozen with meat sauce	8 oz. 7½ oz.	29.7 43
Lemon juice, fresh	1 lemon	4
Mango, fresh	1 medium	33.6
Matzoh meal	1 cup	94
Mayonnaise	1 tbsp.	0.2
Milk, condensed, sweetened	1 cup	166
Milk, evaporated	1 cup	24
Milk, whole, skim, or buttermilk	1 cup	12
Oil		0
Onion, raw, chopped	½ cup	7.5
Papaya	4 oz.	11.3
Peanuts	½ cup, shelled	13
Peanut butter	1 tbsp.	2–4
Pecans	½ cup, shelled	7.9
Pimiento, canned	4 oz.	6.6
Pizza, home baked, with cheese	4 oz.	32
Popcorn, plain	2 cups	10.7

Food	Amount	Carbohydrate Content (Grams)
Potato chips	1 oz.	14
Raisins, whole	½ cup	55.7
Ravioli, canned, beef	1 cup	28.3
Relish, hot-dog	1 tbsp.	5
Sardines, canned in oil	3 oz.	0
Sesame seeds, dry, whole	1 oz.	6.1
Soybean curd	4 oz.	2.7
Soy milk	8 oz.	4.3
Succotash, frozen	½ cup	19
Sugar	1 tbsp.	12.1
Sunflower seeds, hulled	1 oz.	5.6
Sweet potato, peeled	1 medium	38
Tomato, fresh	1 medium	7
Tomato juice	½ cup	5.2
Tomato paste	6 oz.	31
Tomato purée	1 cup	22
Tomato sauce	1 cup	20
Vegetable juice cocktail, canned	4 oz.	4.1
Vegetables, mixed, frozen	½ cup	12

4

EXERCISE: ESSENTIAL FOR DIABETICS

Better to hunt in Fields, for Health unbought,
than fee the doctor for a nauseous Draught.
The Wise, for Cure, on exercise depend;
God never made his Work, for Man to mend.
—JOHN DRYDEN

You have to have buried yourself up to your eyebrows and worn earplugs not to know that exercise is good for you. Everyone in America today seems to be involved in fitness programs of one variety or another, from yoga to running, and that includes plenty of diabetics. We all know now that regular vigorous exercise strengthens the cardiovascular system, lowers "bad" LDL cholesterol levels in the blood while raising the "good" HDL, tones your muscles, improves your circulation, lowers your blood pressure and heart rate, promotes a sense of well-being, and burns off excess weight.

That is quite a list of benefits, but exercise is especially good medicine for most diabetics who, because they have a special tendency toward overweight, poor circulation, high cholesterol and triglycerides, elevated blood pressure, blood clots and accelerated arteriosclerosis, need all the help they can get.

But exercise does even more for you. It can actually help keep your diabetes under control and lower your insulin requirements. In fact, in an eleven-year study of 652 type 2 diabetics, UCLA researchers found that regular exercise and a stringent diet were enough in many cases to keep blood sugar in check without medication. In other words, enough to lower their glucose level to the nondiabetic range so they did not require oral medication or insulin injections.

Did you hear the one about the waltzing mice? In an experiment with mice that were bred to become diabetics, researchers found that if a certain gene was implanted that made the mice stay on the move every waking moment, they did not develop diabetes no matter what they ate. In other words, he who eats and runs away, lives to eat another day. Diabetics should take the hint and keep moving, too.

INVISIBLE INSULIN

Exercise has been called "invisible insulin," and that's just what it is. The more exercise you get, if you are in good health, the less insulin you are likely to require and the more stable your diabetes will probably be. Besides, you can eat more when you exercise more. As one of the early diabetologists once said, "through the sweat of your brow you can earn your bread."

Exercise lowers the level of glucose circulating in your bloodstream. Muscles use glucose as their fuel, first consuming whatever is in the blood, then calling on the liver to deliver more from its stores of glycogen, using it faster than it can be produced. Unless this is carried to an extreme, it is obviously a fine feature for a diabetic who has the chronic problem of glucose disposal. There is evidence, too, that this improved glucose tolerance tends to last for a number of hours after exercise, sometimes even through the next day.

Scientists at the Mayo Clinic suggest frequent exercise, perhaps every other day, rather than isolated spurts of activity, for middle-aged or older diabetics. That's because the boost in sensitivity to insulin may not last more than four or five days among people over the age of forty. The recommendation for persistent insulin benefit is to exercise at least every other day, working up to 40 minutes or more of brisk walking five days a week.

Others experts recommend 30 minutes of moderate-intensity exercise on most days of the week, or at least 150 minutes a week as sufficient to develop or maintain a proper fitness level. Still others advise 30 minutes a day to prevent weight gain, or 45 to 60 minutes a day to encourage weight loss. Take your choice.

And how about this recommendation: It's easy to fit half an hour of exercise into your day if you walk the dog briskly 10 minutes every morning, walk around for 10 minutes during your lunch break, and spend another 10 minutes taking a snappy walk or run with Fido before dinner.

EXERCISE BENEFITS THE BRAIN

The brain benefits from exercise just like the rest of the body. People who exercise in middle age are far less likely to develop Alzheimer's and other types of dementia, even many years later, according to researchers at the Karolinka Institute in Stockholm who monitored the exercise habits of nearly 1,500 patients age sixty-five or older for thirty-five years and reported their findings in 2005.

Be sure, however, to check your blood-glucose level before you start doing heavy physical exercise. If your sugar level is high, over 250 or 270 mgs percent before you begin, call off your plans. Your sugar may rise even higher rather than decrease.

With exercise, insulin is also more readily taken up by the body's cells because of an increase in both insulin sensitivity and the actual number of receptors on target cells in muscle, fat, and liver tissue. A study at Yale University Medical Center demonstrated a 30 percent rise in insulin sensitivity among a group of subjects after a six-week program of daily physical training.

A fifteen-year survey of about 3,700 adults with type 2 diabetes, ages twenty-five to seventy-four, was made by the National Public Health Institute in Finland and reported in 2005. It found that those who participated in high levels of physical activity had a 33 percent lower risk of death by heart disease, and those who engaged in moderate exercise showed a 17 percent drop compared to the most sedentary participants.

If you are ready for another documented reason to get exercise, here it is: regular physical activity can reduce your risk of developing the diabetic eye changes called retinopathy and other vascular diabetic complications. Many diabetics have an abnormal tendency toward "sticky" blood platelets, platelets that clump together and form clots. Research at the University of California Medical Center in San Francisco found that, for both type 1 diabetics and normal individuals, there is a significant drop in this stickiness with exercise, an effect that tends to last many hours.

Other researchers who measured the biochemical response to a blockage of veins in healthy adults before and after they participated in a ten-week conditioning program confirmed that regular vigorous exercise improves the ability to dissolve blood clots.

Caution: If you already have retinopathy, this may be another story and vigorous exercise may not be wise. Be especially cautious if you lift weights—never lift them above eye level (see Chapter 10).

A BALANCING ACT

Diabetes control is always a balancing act between intake (food), which must contain enough glucose to fuel the body, and outgo (bodily functions and exercise, perhaps aided by insulin or oral agents). Your doctor always tries to determine how active you are before deciding on the amount of medication you must take. If you don't exercise, you'll need less food and/or more medication than someone in exactly the same medical situation who exercises.

To make this balancing act work (and to keep life simple), it is always best to get approximately the same amount of exercise every day. That way you will know just how much medication you need to take, as well as what to eat. Otherwise, you must make constant adjustments.

But if you are a working person, you probably sit at a desk most of the week and do your exercise on weekends, or maybe you only get out to run or bike or walk every few days. In this case, you have to plan ahead, one day at a time. Some people have two different diets, one for sedentary days, another for active days. If they take insulin, they sometimes inject different amounts as well. Unless you are spilling a lot of sugar (never a good idea), you always run the risk, if you're on insulin, of an insulin reaction when you exercise. This is the number one concern of diabetic athletes.

If you don't take insulin, life is obviously a whole lot easier. First, you don't have to be so careful about eating on time. Second, after you have burned up your sugar you will have less extraneous insulin in your bloodstream to cause a reaction. Even if you take oral medication, reactions won't be a problem for you. Oral medication is not oral insulin, and it is extremely rare for people who don't

take insulin to have insulin shock unless they are very ill
and debilitated, haven't eaten at all for a long period of
time, or have taken a drug that, in combination with
some oral agents, can drop your blood sugar too low.

AVOIDING REACTIONS

Let's face it, if you take insulin and your diabetes is in
good control—which should always be your goal—you
may have to experience an occasional insulin reaction.
This is preferable to constant high blood sugar, which
will eventually take its toll on your body (see Chapter
10). Ideally, you are taking enough insulin to cover your
food and your activities and keep your sugar level normal. When you exercise more than usual, you burn off
extra glucose and may become hypoglycemic unless you
take precautionary measures.

First of all, check your blood sugar before you start
exercising to see if it is too low. If it is, have a snack.
Check again when you've finished your session, and then
again a couple of hours later, to be sure it is in the normal range. Sometimes exercise-induced hypoglycemia
lasts for many hours, sometimes even for another day.
Don't drink alcohol right before and after exercise, and
avoid hot tubs, saunas, and steam rooms because they
too can trigger another big drop in blood sugar. And
don't drive anywhere until you're back to normal.

On a day when you are going to exercise heavily, you
must plan ahead. Either take less insulin or eat more
food, or both. This is something you must work out
with your own doctor, because everyone's requirements
are different; usually an insulin reduction of about 20
percent works out satisfactorily if it is combined with an
increase in protein and carbohydrate. Don't ever try to

make adjustments without your doctor's advice as well as constant blood tests to be sure you are not going from one blood-sugar extreme to the other.

Let's take an example. You plan to run this morning. You test your blood and it is normal or low.

If you take Regular and NPH in combination, reduce your Regular dose by 20 percent (if your doctor agrees), or if it is a small dose omit the Regular insulin and at breakfast eat 10 to 20 *extra* grams of carbohydrate *plus* some protein that will slowly convert to carbohydrate in a few hours.

If you take only NPH insulin, cut back a few units and increase your food.

When you decide to do your heavy physical activity in the afternoon, remember that the intermediate-acting insulin peaks around 3 P.M. You probably should reduce your NPH dose that morning by 20 percent or by whatever amount you and your doctor have decided works best for you.

If you take Lantus or Levemir at night and you know you'll be very active the next morning, it is a good idea to reduce your dose by a few units the night before. Or if you plan strenuous exercise and take two doses of Lantus or Levemir a day—at night and again in the morning—plus fast-acting insulin such as Humulog, NovoLog, or Apidra before meals, then try reducing both morning doses by a few units.

SOME ALTERNATIVE ARRANGEMENTS

• For some people, a more workable plan is to take the usual dose of insulin, then to add more food to make up the difference, especially when activities aren't predictable in advance.

• For overweight diabetics, lowering the insulin intake is probably better than adding calories. This way, you can lose weight at the same time.

• Now, suppose you plan to exercise today and when you test your blood you see an elevated blood-sugar level. If it isn't excessively high, you can use the exercise to help your insulin bring down the sugar. Take your normal dose and eat a little less carbohydrate at the meal before you start off.

• If, on the other hand, you are going to be exercising *really* rigorously, the recommendation is to take your full complement of food and assume the exercise itself will act like extra insulin.

• Exception: if you wake up with diabetic acidosis, or near-acidosis, exercise will aggravate your situation. If your sugar level is up to around 250 or 270 mgs, forget your plans. That's easy, because you won't feel like going through with them anyway.

SNACKING FOR SAFETY

A carbohydrate or protein-and-carbohydrate snack about a half hour before the run or the game is recommended if your blood sugar is normal or low. Again, you must work this out with your doctor or by trial and error.

Sometimes planning ahead isn't enough. Perhaps you'll need some quick-acting carbohydrate *during* your exercise. If the tennis match goes into the fourth or fifth set and you still haven't won, your breakfast or lunch plus a snack may not be enough to get you through. Stop for a few seconds, take out some of your emergency rations, which you must *always* carry with you, and have a snack to boost your blood sugar. If you're playing golf, plan to snack at the ninth hole. Don't wait for the eleventh or twelfth or you may be sorry.

For most people, a small amount of carbohydrate about every 20 minutes during very hard exercise is sufficient. You'll soon get a sense of how much you need, and how often. A pitcher for the old Boston Braves had it all worked out in peanuts. If he had to throw more pitches or give up more hits than he'd anticipated, he ate extra peanuts based on the number of balls thrown at the plate.

Along with carbohydrate to counteract low blood sugar, you must also replace lost fluids. Your body needs the fluid you have lost through sweating. Drink plenty of water. Avoid the commercial electrolyte glucose drinks—they are too concentrated for you and may raise your blood sugar too quickly.

BE READY FOR ANYTHING

Don't wait for a warning that an insulin reaction is coming; sometimes there is none. Anticipate. If you're a newcomer to diabetes or exercise, remember you will soon be able to tell when it is time for a booster. Suppose you are playing baseball. Instead of striking out and sitting down on the bench in your usual fashion, you make a three-base hit. Now you've got to make a mad sprint around the bases. Or you're late for the 5:45 train and run a few blocks to catch it. You haven't planned on it and so you have not adjusted your food or your medication. This is the time to pull out those emergency rations from your pocket and eat them.

Just a *small* amount of food will do the job. If you need more in 15 minutes, take a little more (see Chapter 8). Many people panic and overshoot the mark, taking too much sugar to ward off a reaction. While they may have made the train or won the ball game, now they have to pay the price of very high sugar that may be harder to cope with than the other extreme.

It's best to exercise *after* a meal, though obviously you should give yourself time to do a little digesting first. After you have eaten, your blood-sugar level is on the rise. Before a meal, it may be very low. For most people who take insulin, the best time to exercise is in the morning after breakfast. But if you can only work out in midafternoon, remember that your NPH is peaking at that moment. Besides considering lowering your morning dose, be sure to have a snack first and be on the lookout for reactions.

CHECK IT OUT

When you are on insulin, it's essential to test your blood for an up-to-the-minute report before going out to do heavy exercise. If it tests low before you even begin, you will know you need some carbohydrate for sure.

If you'll be driving yourself home after a tennis match or an aerobic stint, check your blood before you get into the car. If you've been driving more than a half hour, pull over and check your blood sugar. If necessary, have a snack, which, of course, you always keep handy in your pocket or glove compartment. You are much more likely to get where you're going if you take precautions.

THE IMPORTANCE OF SHAPING UP

When you first start an exercise program, don't leap right in and go at it strenuously. Work up to it slowly, after a discussion with your doctor (yes, yes, yes, talk to your doctor even about this), and if you are over forty, you need a cardiovascular assessment before you begin.

There's probably no reason you can't participate in any kind of sports or exercise like anyone else, but you must give yourself time to adjust your food and medication requirements and to get your body in condition. Sudden strenuous exercise is dangerous for anyone, but especially for you.

For most people, aerobic exercise, the kind that makes your heart and lungs work harder, is recommended at least three times a week for at least thirty minutes a day. To burn calories and increase muscle tone, your desired heart rate should be 85 percent of 220 minus your age. Avoid high-impact activities if you have eye or nerve damage, but walking, swimming, and biking are good choices for almost everyone.

EXERCISE MAY NOT BE FOR YOU

Though everyone needs a certain amount of physical activity to burn calories and sugar, vigorous exercise is not recommended for some diabetics. That's why it is always imperative to consult your physician before you set out to be an athlete. If your diabetes is in poor control, you may do yourself more harm than good. Studies have shown that, rather than lowering blood glucose as in well-controlled people, prolonged strenuous exercise may *raise* your sugar level as well as increase the production of ketones. So it may actually aggravate your diabetes.

Exercise may also be contraindicated for you if you have certain diabetic complications. Obviously, foot or leg problems may be one of these (again, this is individual—sometimes exercise is very helpful in promoting circulation in these areas). Others may include, for example, retinopathy, because rising blood pressure during exercise may cause hemorrhaging; kidney disease, because exercise increases albumin excretion; heart disease, because of the danger of overexerting (exercise may be just what you need, however, but only under medical supervision and with a program tailor-made for you).

CHOOSING THE RIGHT INJECTION SITE

One simple way to help avoid hypoglycemia (insulin reaction) when you exercise is to remember that *where* you inject yourself can make all the difference. If you will be using your legs—running, biking—then you should not inject your insulin in a leg that day because it will be absorbed more rapidly, perhaps precipitating a reaction. If you will be using your right arm, choose your left for your injection today. Remember, too, that injections in the arms or abdomen—if these are not your customary sites—can also absorb much more quickly than those in the legs. So you may have to reduce your dose by a few units, unless your sugar is high, if you make a switch to these new areas.

As a general rule, however, it is always best to take your shots in one area, such as the abdomen, because the results will tend to be more uniform. The newer insulins, however, seem to absorb equally well from any site.

BEWARE THE "MONDAY SYNDROME"

"The housewife who cleans the house on Sunday may have an insulin reaction on Monday." In other words, after some really heavy exercise, your insulin requirements may remain at a lower level the following day

while your muscles replenish their supplies of glucose
and your liver stocks up on glycogen again. You may
need to eat more (or take less insulin) to compensate for
this. Again, individual judgment is required here because it is true for some diabetics and not others.

KEEP A WEATHER WATCH

Your food and insulin needs may also be affected by heat
or cold, either of which can make you burn more energy
and therefore become more susceptible to a reaction.

GET A BUDDY

It is never smart to be alone when you are doing the kind
of exercise that may produce a reaction. Activities such
as skiing, running, swimming, or sailing can be dangerous if no one is around when you need help. Anyway,
they are more fun when you have company, so find
yourself a fellow athlete. Let that person know you have
diabetes and explain what to do if you have a reaction
(see Chapter 8).

CHECK OUT YOUR WARDROBE

The right gear is important for any sport or exercise, but
when you are a diabetic you especially want to avoid
certain things—overheating, sore feet, sunburn. Wear
the proper shoes for your sport, making sure they fit
well, do not rub, and are well cushioned. Under them,
wear absorbent heavy-duty socks that fit smoothly. No
lumps. No holes. Or wear socks made especially for dia-

betics, which have no irritating seams. Check your feet every night for blisters or other injuries. Don't exercise with feet that look like trouble. Watch all of this because diabetics are particularly susceptible to potentially serious circulatory problems (see Chapter 10). Wear layers of clothes so you can shed some if you need to.

DANGER: FROSTBITE

When participating in winter sports, remember to take special care of your hands and feet. If you have poor circulation, this can be vitally important—frostbite is not what you need. Wear a warm hat, lined gloves, wool socks, and warm boots. Go inside frequently and check your fingers and toes (as well as your face and ears) to be sure there is no change in color or sensation. Frostbite means a quick trip to the doctor. Don't try to deal with it yourself. If a doctor isn't immediately available, however, immerse the frostbitten area in lukewarm (never hot) water or cover it with a clean cloth or blanket until you see the doctor.

REMEMBER YOUR SUPPLIES

Be sure whatever you are wearing has pockets, because you will need a place to stash concentrated quick-acting sugar, glucose gel or tablets, or a small carbohydrate snack, along with your identification card. If you have no pockets, stash a few glucose tablets in your socks just above your ankle. That's where surgeons like to keep their wallets in the operating room. Some people like to wear a belt designed to hold sugar or candy, the card, and even a small plastic bottle for a drink. Others hang a plastic pouch of supplies on their belts. Of course, if you are going to be in one place, such as a tennis court, you can carry your goodies in a separate bag.

NO ALCOHOLIC CELEBRATIONS

Many people feel that a nip of wine, a shot of whiskey, or a few beers on the ski slopes or at the finish of a tough bout on the playing field is only what they deserve. But athletics and alcohol don't mix, especially for diabetics. Exercise lowers your blood sugar. At the same time, alcohol inhibits the release of glucose from the liver in response to that low blood sugar, and so it may have quite a different effect than you expect. Right now, you need the glucose from your liver to fuel your brain and replenish your supply. If you drink, you may have an insulin reaction then and there. Give up the nip for a little protein or carbohydrate.

HOW MUCH IS ENOUGH?

Here's how much exercise you should do five days a week to burn off about 2,000 calories:

Swimming	30 minutes a day
Aerobic exercise	40 minutes a day
Tennis (singles)	57 minutes a day
Running	30 minutes a day
Walking (4.4 mph)	60 minutes a day

If you get an hour's lunch break, eat for 45 minutes and take a 15-minute brisk walk. You could lose 1,000 to 1,500 calories a month—4 to 5 pounds a year. Thirty-five hundred calories is equal to about one pound of weight.

5

TAKING ORAL AGENTS

Swallowing a couple of small pills every day is much more appealing and less complicated than giving yourself insulin injections. So if the oral hypoglycemic drugs work for you, consider yourself lucky. There is little need to worry about reactions, no concern about always eating on time, no fuss and muss with needles and syringes and measuring out insulin.

The oral hypoglycemic agents are not for every diabetic because they require that your pancreas has functioning islet cells capable of secreting insulin. Type 1 or IDDM diabetics cannot benefit from them. The typical person for whom oral agents work well is a "mild" type 2 diabetic who would probably require less than 40 units of insulin, and was diagnosed after the age of forty or fifty.

Insulin can't be given orally because it would be destroyed by digestive enzymes. The oral agents are not insulin. They are not even related to insulin. Instead, they are synthetic drugs that lower your blood sugar. Some of them stimulate your pancreas to recognize that the glucose level of your blood has risen and to release the appropriate insulin in response. Others lower blood sugar by inhibiting the release of glucose from the liver or increase the effectiveness of your own or injected insulin by inhibiting the effects of glucagon, which counteracts insulin.

Still others inhibit the absorption of carbohydrate,

stimulate the pancreas to make new beta cells, or keep those you already have from dying. Today, in fact, there is a huge number of oral drugs, as well as injectables other than insulin, which will lower your blood sugar. Your doctor will have to figure out which drug, or what combination of drugs, does the best job for you.

The drugs most commonly used today are the sulfonylureas, especially Glucotrol, Glucotrol XL, and Amaryl. Sulfonylureas, the first oral antidiabetic drugs, were discovered by a French scientist who was looking for an effective antibiotic and found that a type of sulfa drug had the secondary effect of lowering blood sugar by stimulating the production and release of insulin from the beta cells. Similar to the sulfonylureas are Prandin and Starlix, two drugs that have no sulfa in their composition but can do the same.

In addition to the sulfonylureas, several other kinds of oral hypoglycemic agents have become very popular because they do such an excellent job for people with mild type 2 diabetes and those at risk for it. Metformin (Glucophage) tops the list, with acarbose (Precose) and miglitol (Glyset) in second place. Both lower blood sugar without raising the insulin level. Metformin decreases the liver's capacity for producing glucose, while acarbose delays the absorption of carbohydrate in the digestive system.

Actos and Avandia, known as glitazones or TZDs, are other oral medications that lower insulin resistance, while a whole new class of insulin enhancers called incretins, currently administered only by injection but soon to be taken by mouth, have been added to the list of drugs for type 2 diabetics. You'll read more about these agents later in this chapter.

Theoretically, since none of the newer oral agents increase the amount of insulin in your bloodstream, they may be healthier for you than insulin or the sulfonylureas. It's best not to have excessive insulin circulating in your body because it can result in increased blood pressure, atherosclerosis, and weight gain.

ARE ORAL AGENTS SAFE?

According to all current evidence, oral hypoglycemic agents do *not* increase your chances of heart attack, as was once feared.

Many years ago, an extensive eight-year study called the University Group Diabetes Program linked the oral hypoglycemic agents with an increased risk of death from heart disease. The study's conclusions caused many doctors to stop prescribing the pills and replace them with insulin injections if their patients' diabetes could not be controlled with diet.

These claims have now been denied by both the American Diabetic Association and the American Medical Association. Doctors who have been prescribing the oral hypoglycemics for over thirty years have found no increase in heart disease among their patients. Nor have other studies found any differences in the incidence of heart attacks.

As a result, all diabetologists today recommend the oral hypoglycemics for appropriate patients, because these drugs present far fewer problems than insulin injections do. If you are a diabetic who cannot control your diabetes with diet alone, and can achieve a normal blood-sugar level without having to take a shot every day and without having to be concerned with insulin reactions and rigid eating schedules, it definitely makes good sense to choose the pills.

There are limits to how much of any one drug can be taken, however, so when the maximum dose of a drug isn't enough to keep blood glucose levels in the desired range, another drug can be added, perhaps even combined in the same pill.

THE SULFONYLUREAS

The sulfonylureas, the first oral agents for diabetics, help to increase insulin production in the pancreas. They include glipizides (Glucotrol, Glucotrol XL); gliburides (Micronase, Glynase, and DiaBeta); and glimepirides (Amaryl). An early oral drug, chloropropamide (Diabinese), is used only rarely today, as are Orinase, Glynase, Micronase, and Tolinase. The sulfonylureas are taken usually once or twice a day before meals.

Glucotrol and *Glucotrol XL, Glynase,* and *Amaryl* are the strongest of the oral agents today and probably the most commonly prescribed of the sulfonylureas. They are all mildly diuretic. The glipizides and the glyburides work by stimulating the pancreas to release more insulin after meals and by reducing the production of glucose from the liver. Amaryl, prescribed more and more today, is a sulfonylurea but uses different pathways to increase the efficiency of the body's available insulin. It works in concert with exercise and gives you less risk of hypoglycemia.

THE BIGUANIDE METFORMIN (GLUCOPHAGE)

This class of oral antidiabetic drug is very popular today and for good reason: It has improved the lives of many mild diabetics and has several advantages over the sulfonylureas. It is metformin (sold under the brand name Glucophage), available in Europe and Canada for over 30 years before its approval in the United States in 1995.

This drug is a biguanide, a class of drugs derived from a plant called goat's rue or French lilac and used in the Middle Ages for medicinal purposes. This author was among the first to discover that it lowers cholesterol, triglycerides, and weight as well as blood sugar.

Unlike the sulfonylureas, metformin (Glucophage) does not work by stimulating insulin secretion. Instead, it suppresses the liver's production of glucose by up to 75 percent, reducing levels circulating in the bloodstream. At the same time, it increases your own insulin's ability to metabolize sugar up to 29 percent. In other words, it is a glucose-disposal drug.

When used alone, metformin almost never causes hypoglycemia or low blood sugar although it may when combined, as it frequently is, with a sulfonylurea or insulin. It reduces LDL and triglyceride levels and modestly increases HDL, just what the doctor ordered. Because it controls blood sugar by decreasing the amount of insulin in the bloodstream, it may decrease the risk of arteriosclerosis. Besides, it reduces blood pressure in hypertensive and nonhypertensive diabetics, lowers platelet aggregation, and improper arterial dilatation. Best of all, unlike sulfonylureas or insulin, it does not cause weight gain and may, in fact, help you lose a few pounds.

Taken before meals in doses of 500 to 2,500 mgs spaced out over a day, metformin (Glucophage) sometimes produces side effects—nausea, diarrhea, metallic taste—which usually dissipate within a couple of weeks. If they don't, this drug is not for you. Nor is it for you if you have liver or kidney disease, metabolic acidosis, or congestive heart failure. And it is not recommended for alcoholics, children, or pregnant women. If you have an IVP (intravenous pyelogram) or a CT scan with contrast, you must stop taking it for two days after the procedure.

According to the United Kingdom Prospective Diabetes Study in 1998, this was the only diabetic drug shown to reduce the incidence of fatal heart attacks when used alone.

An extended-release form of this oral drug is Glucophage XR, which is taken just once a day with the evening meal and may be easier on your gastrointestinal tract. Metformin also comes in a liquid form called Riomet.

This highly respected drug is often used together with insulin as well as other oral drugs and is even available in several premixed formulations.

ALPHA-GLUCOSIDASE INHIBITORS

Other oral agents are acarbose (Precose) and miglitol (Glyset), starch-blocking drugs that are usually used in combination with insulin or one of the sulfonylureas and probably are most appropriate for diabetics who aren't quite making it with other medications.

Precose and Glyset work by delaying the digestion and absorption of carbohydrates (sugars and starches) in the small intestines. The carbohydrates continue farther down the intestines, where they encounter L cells that produce GLP1, a substance that inhibits the liver's production of glucagon that, in turn, counteracts the effects of insulin. The overall effect is to diminish peaks in blood-sugar levels after meals.

Not as potent as metformin or the sulfonylureas, Precose and Glyset are taken with the first bite of a meal and may be used on their own or in combination with other oral agents or insulin. They have a few gastrointestinal effects, most noticeably flatulence and diarrhea, which usually diminish over time. They should always be taken with a meal and are not recommended for those with kidney disease or intestinal problems. If you weigh less than 130 pounds, don't take a dose of Precose greater than 150 mg a day. Glyset, however, may be taken in the standard dose regardless of your weight.

THIAZOLIDINEDIONES (TZDS) OR GLITAZONES

Actos (pioglitazone) and Avandia (rosiglitazone), members of the drug class known as glitazones or thiazolidinediones (TZDs), are oral antidiabetic drugs designed to help poorly controlled type 2 diabetics make better use of the insulin they produce naturally or acquire through injections. Called "insulin sensitizers," they lower insulin resistance by increasing the absorption of sugar by muscle tissue and, in high doses, reduce the amount of sugar released by the liver. Rezulin (troglitazone), the first drug available in this class, is no longer on the market because of adverse effects on the liver.

The newer TZDs, Actos and Avandia, are excellent drugs that help preserve the lives of pancreatic beta cells by preventing their destruction and, at the same time, increasing their numbers. The TZDs may also prevent clots and therefore heart attacks. And finally, they lower the levels of both LDL cholesterol and triglycerides.

A big plus: These drugs, taken alone, never lower your blood sugar below normal, so you needn't worry about insulin reactions. However, if they are supplemented by insulin or one of the sulfonylureas, that advantage is wiped out.

An even bigger plus: Actos and Avandia may help prevent Alzheimer's disease, which type 2 diabetics are twice as likely to develop. In a study sponsored by the National Institute on Aging, people taking these oral drugs cut their risk of Alzheimer's by 20 percent over those taking insulin.

The negatives of the TZDs include possible weight gain and fluid retention, especially in the ankles, and so they are not recommended for anyone who has heart failure or who already suffers from edema.

In addition, Avandia and Avandamet (a combination of Avandia and metformin) have been accused of causing diabetic eye complications in rare cases. If you notice any changes in your vision, such as blurriness, tell your doctor and be sure to see an opthalmologist whose specialty is retinopathy.

Some physicians hesitate to prescribe them for elderly diabetics, but if tests show that the liver and kidneys are functioning properly, there's no reason to deny older patients the good things that these drugs can provide for them.

Avandia and Actos are classified as "gamma" TZDs. Another variety, "alpha" TZDs, improves lipid metabolism. Combinations of the two will soon be on the market. The first such drug to be developed, however, called Pargluva (muraglitazar), turned out to have serious side effects and is not available.

MEGLITINIDES

Prandin (repatlinide) and Starlix (nateglinide) are similar to the sulfonylureas but work faster and do not last as long, so there is less chance of developing hypoglycemia. Both are used mostly by very mild diabetics whose blood sugars are just over normal. The drugs are taken right before a meal because they stimulate the release of insulin *only* in the presence of carbohydrates.

Prandin and Starlix can make your life as a diabetic very easy—you can carry them with you and take them just before you sit down to eat. Both induce the pancreas

ORAL ANTIDIABETIC AGENTS

Drug Class	Trade Name	Generic Name	Size
Sulfonylureas	Orinase*	Tolbutamide	500 mg
	Tolinase*	Tolazamide	100 mg, 250 mg, 500 mg
	Diabinese*	Chlorpropa-mide	100 mg, 250 mg
	DiaBeta	Glyburide	1.25 mg, 2.5 mg, 5 mg
	Micronase*	Glyburide	1.25 mg, 2.5 mg, 5 mg
	Glynase Prestab*	Glyburide	1.5 mg, 3 mg, 6 mg
	Glucotrol	Glipizide	5 mg, 10 mg
	Glucotrol XL	Glipizide	5 mg, 10 mg
Biguanides	Glucophage	Metformin	500 mg, 800 mg, 1,000 mg
	Glucophage XR	Metformin (long-acting)	500 mg, 850 mg
	Riomet	Metformin (liquid)	500 mg per teaspoon
	Glimepiride	Amaryl	1 mg, 2 mg, 4 mg
Alpha-Glucosidase Inhibitors	Precose	Acarbose	25 mg, 50 mg, 100 mg
	Glyset	Miglitol	25 mg, 50 mg, 100 mg
Meglinitides	Prandin	Repaglinide	0.5 mg, 1 mg, 2 mg
	Starlix	Nateglinide	60 mg, 120 mg
TZDs (Glitazones)	Avandia	Rosiglitazone	4 mg and 8 mg
	Actos	Pioglitazone	15 mg, 30 mg, 45 mg

*These first-generation oral agents are rarely used today.

to produce enough insulin to deal with your blood sugar after a meal.

These drugs can be taken alone if you are a mild diabetic, or with other drugs such as metformin (Glucophage) or acarlose (Precose) if you require more action.

TAKING A COMBINATION OF DRUGS

If an oral agent doesn't control your blood glucose effectively, you can try a different one, add a second oral agent, or take two oral drugs combined in the same pill. For example, Glucovance combines metformin (Glucophage) with a glyburide, Avandamet mixes metformin with Avandia, and Metaglip mixes it with Actos.

COMBI.NATION ORAL AGENTS

Trade Name	Generic Name	Size
Glucovance	Glyburide and Metformin	1.25mg/250mg, 2.5mg/500mg, 5mg/500mg
Avandamet	Rosiglitazone and Metformin	1mg/500mg 2mg/500mg 4mg/500mg 2mg/1,000mg 4mg/1,000mg
Avandaryl	Avandia and Amaryl	4 mg/1 mg 4mg/2 mg 4 mg/4 mg
Metaglip	Metformin and Glipizide	2.5mg/250mg 2.5mg/500mg 5mg/500mg
Glumetza	Amaryl and Metformin	500 mg, 1,000mg
ActoplusMet	Metformin and Actos	15 mg/500mg, 15mg/850mg

INCRETINS: A NEW CLASS OF DRUGS

Once again, innovative drugs promise to transform the lives of type 2 diabetics. A brand-new class of drugs—about to come on the market at the time of this writing—is based on the physiology of the gila monster, a poisonous lizard whose saliva contains a substance called GLP-1 that incapacitates its prey by dramatically reducing blood sugar.

This same substance is made in the human digestive tract and helps stimulate insulin production after meals. It is accompanied by a second substance—DPP-4—that quickly destroys the GLP-1. Because, just as it does for the gila monster, human GLP-1 can reduce blood sugar, researchers looked for a way to extend its life so it could be used for blood-sugar control in diabetics. They created a synthetic version of DPP-4 that, combined with GLP-1, increases its ability to remain in the body long enough to do the job.

The resulting drugs protect the life span of the insulin-producing beta cells by preventing their destruction and perhaps encouraging the formation of new cells. This could be a godsend for mild diabetics who may even "lose" their disease if enough new cells are produced. The TZDs also protect the beta cells but tend to cause weight gain.

WHAT'S THEIR PROBLEM?

The first-generation incretins, Byetta (exanatide) and Liraglutide, must be taken by injection, not to everyone's liking, although oral versions are in development. They sometimes cause unacceptable nausea, at least for a few weeks or months, and there have been no long-term studies to determine if there will be deleterious effects over the years.

The good news is that the incretins also encourage weight loss, sometimes dramatically. They delay gastric emptying, increase satiety, slow the release of glucagon from the liver, and stimulate insulin secretion—all good things for type 2 diabetics. These drugs are used primarily by mild type 2s to supplement oral agents such as the sulfonylureas or metformin, although they may eventually be used as stand-alone drugs.

The best feature of the incretins is that they work *only* when blood glucose levels are high, shutting off when the sugar gets as low as 90 mg/dl. This means that, on their own, they won't lower sugar below a safe level. But if you take them together with one of the sulfonylurea agents, you'll still have to be on the lookout for reactions.

Byetta (exenatide) was the first incretin to be approved by the FDA and is taken by injection before breakfast and dinner. Liraglutide, the next to be developed, requires once-a-day injections. Other drugs still in the pipeline may need to be injected just once a week or even once a month, although they are not expected to be as effective as the daily varieties.

The oral versions of incretins are coming along very soon and they will certainly appeal to people who like pills better than injections. Among them are DPP-IV inhibitors, sitgliptin (Januvia), saxagliptin, and vildagliptin (Galvas). Strangely, the drugs taken by mouth are "weight-neutral," but if you take them with metformin, you may lose weight and improve your glucose numbers, too.

SYMLIN AND ITS VIRTUES

Symlin (pramlintide) is a drug designed to make control easier for type 1 diabetics. A synthetic injectable form of a natural hormone secreted by the pancreas, it is taken *in addition to* insulin when even huge doses of insulin fail to achieve the desired glucose levels.

Symlin blocks the secretion of amylin, a hormone also produced by the pancreas, that diminishes the effects of insulin. Among Symlin's many other virtues, it delays gastric emptying, diminishes the release of glucagon from the liver, prolongs the working lives of the all-important beta cells, and suppresses the appetite.

An important downside is that it increases the likelihood of severe insulin reactions, making it extremely important to monitor your sugar level throughout the day. When you take Symlin, you must reduce your usual insulin dose by half.

DIET IS STILL IMPORTANT

Just because you are taking oral agents instead of insulin does not mean that you are home free. You still cannot eat whatever you like. Hot fudge sundaes are still not an option, at least not very often, nor is too much food of any kind. For any diabetic, diet is the most important part of the therapy. The pills will not transform you into a normal person with a normal pancreas that turns out as much insulin as you need to respond to an overload of sugar.

If you eat too much, you—just like an insulin-dependent diabetic—may end up in the hospital in a coma. Not only that, but if your diabetes is consistently out of control, even to a degree that isn't obvious to you, you are greatly increasing your risk of developing diabetic complications in the future. *Just like an insulin-dependent person, you are a real diabetic.* However, if you maintain your proper weight, eat sensibly, and get enough exercise, it is possible you may no longer need the oral agents and will not be considered diabetic but merely someone with a tendency toward the disease.

Extra pills are not like extra insulin. Many people think if they overdose on food, they can compensate by taking extra pills. They cannot. They will simply go out of control and have high blood sugar, which is just as harmful to them as to any other diabetic. When your fixed maximum effect has been reached, additional pills will do no good.

TALLY YOUR TESTS

You must also test your blood regularly. If you are well controlled, you should make tests twice a day—before breakfast and before bed or before supper. If you are not, test three or four times a day until your sugar is down. Keep a record of the results and take this to your doctor. Together you can decide how to change your diet and/or your activities so you may not have to switch to insulin.

Illnesses, excessive sugar in your diet, less exercise, more stress, etc., can cause you to spill sugar and perhaps acetone. If your sugar is high, always test for acetone in the urine. If acetone is present, confer with your doctor and be aware that you must get your sugar down quickly. A temporary supplement of insulin may be what you need. Going over to insulin during an illness or pregnancy does not make you insulin-dependent. When you no longer need the shots, you can probably return to your former regime.

WHEN YOU ARE SICK

Whenever you have an infection, especially when it is accompanied by a fever, your insulin requirements will rise. That's because not only does your liver release extra glucose as part of the body's defenses against attack but more glucose is formed from protein when you are under stress. Now you may not get enough insulin response from your pill-primed pancreas to handle this increased sugar. If your tests show prolonged high sugars, something must be done to avoid acidosis.

Your doctor will probably suggest, if you normally take only a small amount of oral medication, that you are vigilant about your diet and perhaps raise your dosage to increase the pills' efficiency. When you are already taking your maximum effective dose, however, taking more is not the answer. You have reached your limit of insulin production.

INSULIN, BUT NOT FOREVER

If your blood sugar does not return to normal, you'll need to turn to insulin temporarily, alone or as a supplement. Unless you are an old hand at this, do nothing on your own. Let your doctor make the decisions. Probably 5 to 10 units of fast-acting insulin every two hours will turn the tide.

That is why you must know how to give yourself injections and keep a bottle of fast-acting insulin stored in your refrigerator (replace it when it becomes outdated). Your doctor will tell you how often to take it.

Temporary insulin injections will also be needed by most diabetics on oral agents when they have major surgery. The reason is the same—increased need for insulin during stress. Sometimes, too, you may need insulin injections when you are sick and can't tolerate anything—including your oral agents—by mouth.

Many people think that once they take insulin when they are sick, they must stay on it forever. Not true. You can almost always go back to the oral agents when you recover.

POSSIBLE SIDE EFFECTS OF THE ORAL AGENTS

Once in a while, a diabetic reacts unfavorably to the oral hypoglycemic agents. The possible side effects include nausea and other gastrointestinal problems, fever, skin rashes, itching. If these symptoms do not diminish and then disappear at your lowest possible dosage, the only solution is to try other oral agents, switch over to insulin, or watch your diet more strictly.

MUST YOU WORRY ABOUT REACTIONS?

Hypoglycemic reactions are an *extremely* rare occurrence when you take oral agents because your pancreas is sensitized to respond only to the glucose content of your bloodstream. The insulin does not pour out as soon as you swallow your pills, as it does from an injection, but waits until it is required.

But reactions *are* possible. Too high a dosage, unexpected and very heavy exercise, and consistent insufficiency of food (especially among the elderly, who may not have a sufficient store of glycogen) can all trigger a hypoglycemic reaction. Usually the reaction is mild and easily reversible because your blood sugar does not drop as far or as fast as it would if you were taking insulin. It may make you feel weak, trembly, faint, or headachy.

Very severe reactions can occur, however, and can be much worse than reactions from insulin because they may be sudden, prolonged—perhaps lasting for days—and life-threatening. Although they are sometimes the result of overlapping effects of long-acting oral agents, they are more likely to happen when a diabetic continues to take the pills but does not eat or has a gastrointestinal upset.

Often people think that, because their diabetes responds to the pills and does not require insulin shots, they can be lackadaisical about monitoring their blood sugar. However, they must pay attention, make sure to eat enough food to cover the medication, and check their blood sugar at least twice a day.

WATCH OUT FOR DRUG INTERACTIONS

Sometimes reactions happen for other reasons, too. Liver or kidney disease, for example, can affect the behavior of the oral agents. And so can the interaction of other drugs that are detoxified in the liver, sometimes raising or lowering blood sugar dramatically. These include some antidepressents, antipsychotics, anti-inflammatory agents, beta blockers, corticosteroids, niacin, epilepsy drugs, thiazide diuretics, and some antibiotics.

The popular sulfonylurea Amaryl, for example, should never be taken together, with the antibiotic cipro or other fluoroquinalones because they may trigger a precipitous drop in blood sugar. In addition, no diabetic on oral agents should *ever* take the antibiotic Tequin because it can cause serious cases of very high or very low blood sugar.

You can get in a lot of trouble if you're not aware of these interactions. So don't take chances. Remind your doctor and your pharmacist that you are a diabetic on oral agents—it's amazing how many forget from visit to visit—and ask them if a new drug might affect your sugar control.

DEALING WITH REACTIONS

The treatment for hypoglycemia is always the same—eat some quickly absorbed carbohydrate, along with some protein. Because the hypoglycemia may not be reversed quickly if it is due to overlapping doses of oral agents or disease, your blood sugar should be closely monitored until you're back to normal.

Never skip your meals, and remember to eat extra food if you are going to engage in heavy exercise.

Tell your doctor if you ever have reactions. Because reactions are so rare when you take oral agents, it is most important to know the reason for them.

OTHER DRUG INTERACTIONS

Inderal and other beta blockers, drugs prescribed for hypertension, can block the secretion of insulin and cause the oral agent to be ineffective in some cases.

And very important: the effects of most barbiturates, sedatives, and hypnotics can be seriously prolonged when you take sulfonylurea agents.

WILL THE PILLS EVER BECOME INEFFECTIVE?

For most people, the oral agents continue to do their job indefinitely. Though it was once thought that their effect always diminished after five or ten years, it has been found that only a small percentage of pill-takers have "secondary failure" and must start taking insulin instead.

If your diabetes control seems to be worse, the most likely explanation is that you aren't paying attention to your diet or your need for exercise. Neither pills nor insulin shots will keep you from all the problems of diabetes without proper living habits.

But if you are in the minority whose internal insulin production does diminish with time, a stronger or longer-acting oral agent may help reestablish your control. Not only that, but today, with so many new oral agents available, it is possible to combine these drugs so that they'll do a better job of keeping your blood sugar within normal boundaries.

If this doesn't work, then you must turn to insulin.

ORAL DRUGS PLUS INSULIN

But before switching you over to a total insulin regimen, your diabetic specialist may decide to try BIDS (bedtime insulin/daytime sulfonylureas or other oral agents) in case that's all you need. This means that you take your usual oral agents during the day and add a little insulin at bedtime. This works very well for many people, although it makes insulin reactions more likely, and more and more people are on this regimen.

Keep in mind that reactions when you are on an oral agents—especially when insulin is added—can be very severe, so you must be especially vigilant about your blood-sugar levels. Although reactions when you take oral medication are rare—usually occurring only in cases of severe illness, liver or kidney problems, overlapping medication, age-related frailty, or poor nutrition—you must take them seriously and report them immediately to your doctor.

IF YOU FORGET TO TAKE YOUR DOSE

It is not a good idea to omit your dose of an oral agent and you should *never* stop taking it because you're feeling better, but it isn't a serious matter if you forget to take it only once in a while. That is because you do make some insulin on your own, and a brief period without the agent won't raise your blood sugar to dangerous levels. Simply take your pill when you remember it. If you have gone as long as a whole day without the medication and your blood tests show high sugar, be sure to take your pill immediately. If you are very symptomatic (excessive thirst or urination), call your doctor promptly because you may be heading for acidosis.

6

GOING THE INSULIN ROUTE

All type 1 diabetics, and those type 2s whose blood
sugar cannot be controlled by diet therapy or oral
agents, must take injections of insulin to replace the insulin they no longer make on their own. This means
daily injections, a prospect nobody regards with great
joy. But once you accept them as essential to your
health, they can be managed without turning your life
upside down. Eating on time, sticking to your diet, testing your blood, adjusting your dose, being alert to low
blood sugar as well as high can all become routine parts
of your daily existence that need not always dominate
your thoughts. If insulin therapy is new to you, this may
be hard to believe, but with time and experience you can
learn to go about your business despite being an insulin-
dependent diabetic.

Consider a diabetic's fate before this miracle drug was
discovered. Before 1922, adults who developed diabetes
were lucky to live another ten years, youngsters a few
months. Diet was the only known treatment and starving was the alternative to diabetic coma.

In 1921, Drs. Charles Best and Frederick Banting,
using research by Dr. Moses Barron, extracted a substance from a steer's pancreas and injected it into a diabetic dog, promptly lowering the dog's blood sugar.
With that success, the outlook for diabetics changed

overnight. Drs. Best and Banting next gave the new ex-
tract to each other, waited 24 hours, then injected it into
a twelve-year-old diabetic boy who was near death but
who made a dramatic recovery on a steady regime of
insulin injections. In only a year, Best and Banting and
other scientists developed the techniques for mass-
producing the miracle hormone, literally creating life for
people who previously had been doomed.

TODAY'S INSULIN

Not too long ago, insulin came from the pancreases of
pigs and cattle and its characteristics varied because sometimes more pigs were available and sometimes more cattle. Although the animal insulin became more and more
pure, with most of the contaminants eventually eliminated, some people still had allergic reactions to it.

Today most insulins are synthesized from bacteria or
yeast cells and are biologically identical to human insulin. Genetically altered by gene-splicing, they do an
excellent job and will never be in short supply, as animal
insulin once was, because they are mass produced in factories by very willing workers—bacteria or yeast cells—
who will never go on strike.

The manufactured insulins are combined with other
substances that modify the rate at which they are absorbed and how long they will be effective, so they may
be prescribed according to individual needs. The solubil-
ity of insulin, which determines how quickly it enters the
bloodstream and goes into action, is decided by three
factors: the physical form (amorphous or crystalline)
and, if crystalline, the size of the crystals; the amount of
zinc salts added; and the nature of the buffer solution
holding it.

LANTUS AND LEVEMIR: LONG-ACTING

Among the newest forms of insulin are two long-acting insulins called Lantus (glargine) and Levemir (detemir) that are already among the most commonly used because they do such a remarkably good job for many people. Dubbed the "poor man's insulin pump," these drugs are designed to be taken once or twice a day, at bedtime and perhaps in the morning before breakfast. They replace the older long-lasting insulins because they remain active in the body for approximately 24 hours and do not have "peaks." The durability varies, however. For some people they last only 16 hours, while for others they may be good for 26.

Both of them give you a fairly uniform distribution of insulin throughout the day and night and work well when supplemented by very fast-acting insulins such as Humalog, Novolog, or Apidra that are injected just before or just after a meal and start to function immediately. Because Lantus and Levemir don't and then drop drastically, thereby greatly reducing the possibility of an insulin reaction, they can make your life as a diabetic much easier. What's more, they can be injected anywhere in the body and are less likely than the other insulins to make you gain weight.

Another really big plus is that you don't have to worry about sticking to a rigid schedule of meals. Because the long-acting insulin covers you all day and night, and the fast-acting insulin covers you after a meal, you can be much more relaxed than diabetics have been in the past.

WHAT'S THE NEWS?

Insulin in its present forms must be injected to be effective because taken orally it is destroyed by the digestive enzymes before it reaches the bloodstream. But ever since insulin was discovered, many biotechnology companies have been looking for alternatives to insulin injections. Pretty soon, injections, like the passenger pigeon, will be merely a memory.

The first alternative to injected insulin to come along is very good news for people who hate to inject themselves. This is inhaled insulin, which is designed to replace the quick-acting insulin taken before meals. In January 2006, the FDA approved the use of Exubera, sold by Pfizer. Exubera uses an inhalation device about the size of a flashlight that combines pressurized air with a powered form of insulin powder to create a cloud of insulin that is inhaled through the mouth over several seconds. It is available in 1-mg and 3-mg doses, equivalent to three or eight units of liquid insulin, and is taken just before meals to cover your food. You'll still, however, have to face one or two injections a day of longer-acting insulin.

Other companies are working on their own versions of inhaled insulin. Lilly, for example, is developing a similar product called Alkermes.

A downside of inhaled insulin is that correctly administering it to yourself is rather complicated. Also, it has been found to cause a small decline in lung function in some people, at least at first, making it unsuitable for diabetics with underlying lung disease such as asthma, bronchitis, or emphysema. It is not approved for children and is not recommended for smokers or former smokers who have quit within six months because their lungs might absorb too much of it.

OTHER OUCHLESS OPTIONS

Also under development are other varieties of insulin. One is a pill or capsule that will survive destruction by the enzymes and acids of the digestive tract. Another is an insulin mouth spray to be called Oral-lyn that can be taken just before or after meals because it enters the bloodstream very quickly.

And finally, insulin skin patches may turn out to be the most popular way to go.

A CURE FOR DIABETES?

Not too far in the future, diabetes may actually be cured, making any form of exogenous insulin unnecessary, perhaps by encapsulating insulin-producing pancreatic islet cells and placing them in the abdomen, where they will manufacture the hormone in response to rising blood sugar and turn itself off when the sugar diminishes. In a study reported in 2004 by researchers from twelve medical centers in the U.S. and Canada, 86 people with type 1 diabetes received transplants of islet cells infused through the liver. After six months, 61 percent required no insulin injections because their new islet cells made appropriate amounts of insulin; and after a year, 58 percent required no injections. It's not yet known, however, how long the "cure" will last. We do know that most people require insulin again after about five years, but they don't have severe reactions anymore.

In another trial, conducted from July 2001 to August 2003, doctors gave islet transplants from a single donor pancreas to eight women with type 1 diabetes. Five remained insulin-independent for longer than one year. And in 2005, a Japanese mother ended her daughter's type 1 diabetes, at least short term, by giving her half of her own pancreas. The transplanted cells started producing insulin immediately. In this case, the daughter's diabetes had not been caused by her autoimmunity but by a severe case of pancreatitis, which means that her diabetes is not likely to reoccur.

In the meantime, many scientists believe that stem-cell research has the potential of transforming the lives of diabetics, as well as of people with other diseases, and give it a very high priority. Stem cells promise to become a source of insulin-producing beta cells and may even lead to the prevention or cure of diabetic complications. Adult stem cells may have this ability, but the use of embryonic stem cells—now a hot political issue—is considered a much more likely road to success.

Complete pancreatic transplants are another way to go, with thousands of such procedures having been performed in recent years.

KINDS OF INSULIN

Many varieties and strengths of insulin are now available, and which one or which combination you should take must be sorted out by your doctor. Because type 1 diabetics produce no insulin of their own, they all require daily insulin treatment. Although many type 2 diabetics can control their sugar level with diet, exercise, and oral drugs, about a third of them must add insulin to their daily regimens.

Insulins vary in several ways: the speed at which they work; the length of time they continue to lower blood sugar; when they do or do not "peak" (provide their maximum effects); and their strength.

Following are the categories of insulin on the market

today. Some insulins have been discontinued and others are no longer as popular as they once were, having been superseded by newer varieties. For example, Regular and NPH were the standard for many years and continue to be used by many diabetics who have become accustomed to them. If you are getting good results with them, there is no reason to change. However, most specialists have switched over to the newer drugs because they work with more predictability and cause fewer insulin reactions.

VERY FAST-ACTING INSULIN

The first very fast-acting insulins to come along in many years, Humalog (insulin lispro), NovoLog (insulin aspart), and Apidra (insulin glulisine), have largely supplanted Regular insulin. These "designer" hormones get into the bloodstream almost immediately, mimicking the normal body's response to food, and last 3 to 5 hours.

They work so quickly that they can be injected 15 minutes before a meal. This gives you more flexibility in your eating schedule, even one that changes day to day, because you can take the insulin and promptly sit down and eat. This is a big advantage when you're eating at a restaurant or a dinner party on other people's timetables. But don't make the mistake of taking your shot before you reach your destination, because you may find that the food won't be on the table for another half hour or more. When you know the meal is about to be served, excuse yourself, go to the bathroom or another private spot, and take your dose.

FAST-ACTING INSULIN

Regular insulin is fast-acting clear insulin that takes effect in less than an hour, peaks in 2 to 3 hours, and lasts another couple of hours more. In an emergency, it can be given intravenously for even faster action.

It is rarely used alone on a daily basis, unless you are on a multiple-injection plan, which means that you inject yourself several times a day with small amounts of insulin in response to your blood-sugar level. It is usually combined with other forms for daily use, or used only when you need insulin in a hurry.

INTERMEDIATE-ACTING INSULIN

NPH is a cloudy insulin that lasts 12 to 24 hours in the bloodstream, starts to work about 1 to 1½ hours after injection, and peaks in 8 to 12 hours. This means that it has a small amount of action before lunch and a major effect in midafternoon. The intermediate-acting insulin usually covers you most of the day, including your three meals and the glucose released from your liver during the night.

LONG-ACTING INSULIN

Lantus (glargine) and Levemir (detemir) are long-acting insulins that remain active for up to 24 hours, so one injection a day, most often at bedtime, will usually do the basic job for the whole day. In most cases, they are used in combination with Humalog, NovoLog, or Apidra, very fast-acting insulins that are injected before each meal. Because Lantus and Levemir are slowly absorbed and have no peaks, the worrisome problem of insulin reactions is virtually eliminated, and their effectiveness is equally strong throughout the day.

Sometimes, in an effort to get very tight blood-sugar control, Lantus or Levemir taken at night can be supplemented by a small dose in the morning.

Both of these insulins are *clear* and cannot be combined in the same syringe with any other insulin.

Lantus is available in vials as well as pen injectors, while Levemir comes only in preloaded pens or in 3mL cartridges that can be loaded into most reusable pens.

GUIDE TO INSULINS

Brand Name	Type	Onset	Peak Action
Humulin R	Fast-acting	½ hour	2½–5 hours
Novolin	Fast-acting	½ hour	2½–5 hours
Humalog	Very fast-acting	15 minutes	½–1½ hours
NovoLog	Very fast-acting	10–20 minutes	1–3 hours
Apidra	Very fast-acting	15 minutes	1–3 hours
Humulin N	NPH Intermediate-acting	1½ hours	8–12 hours
Lantus	Long-acting	40 minutes	No peak
Levemir	Long-acting	40 minutes	No peak

PREMIXED COMBINATION INSULINS

Premixed insulin, a combination of two kinds of insulin in one bottle, is a boon to many people because it is less complicated than mixing the insulins in one syringe or taking two injections rather than one. Although it may not be quite as precise as individually tailored doses, it usually provides decent blood-sugar control, especially for milder diabetics.

Premixed Insulin

Humulin 70/30	70% NPH/30% Regular
Novolin 70/30	70% NPH/30% Regular
Humulin 50/50	50% NPH/50% Regular
Humalog 75/25	75% HPS/25% Humalog
NovoLog 70/30	70% NPA/30% NovoLog

INSULIN STRENGTHS

Although insulin used to be available in several strengths (or concentrations), today only U-100 strength is readily available in the United States. All vials sold in the U.S. have 100 units of pure insulin in each milliliter of fluid and are labeled U-100. Each vial contains 1,000 units of fluid and insulin.

If you travel to another country where you may be able to buy only U-40, you can use it, but you must know how to translate from one strength to the other. Just remember that *a unit of insulin is always the same,* no matter what strength you use, and it is always inter-changeable with a unit of any other strength. It has the same potency and blood-sugar-lowering effect. What differs is the amount of solution or liquid in which the insulin is held. One cc of U-40 insulin contains 40 units of insulin. One cc of U-100 contains 100 units of in-sulin. Therefore, one unit of U-40 is larger *in volume* (because of the water content) than a unit of U-100, but the strength of one unit is always the same.

So, *one unit is one unit,* and can be exchanged for one unit of a different strength. BUT you must use a syringe that corresponds with the strength of your insulin (for example, a U-100 syringe for U-100 insulin—both have orange caps) in order to avoid errors.

IN AN EMERGENCY

If you *must* use a syringe that does not correspond to your insulin, then you must make the translation. For example, if you run out of U-100 insulin, and must use U-40 with a U-100 syringe: multiply your usual *volume* (not your units) of U-100 by 2½. This will give you an equivalent U-40 dose. In other words, you need a larger *volume* (2½ times as much) of U-40 to equal the same number of units of U-100 because it is less concentrated.

10 units on U-100 syringe = 4 units of U-40 insulin
20   = 8 units
30   = 12 units
40   = 16 units
50   = 20 units

SYRINGE STRATEGIES

Insulin syringes come in many sizes and shapes and it doesn't matter too much which one you use as long as you are always certain you use one that corresponds with your insulin strength. U-100 syringes are available in 100-unit, 50-unit, and 30-unit sizes, the latter is handy for people who take very small doses. The 100-unit syringe holds 100 units of insulin in 1 cc of liquid. Each line indicates 2 units of insulin. A 50-unit syringe holds 50 units of insulin in 0.5 cc of liquid and *each line marks only 1 unit*. A 30-unit size holds 30 units of insulin in 0.3 cc of liquid and *each line indicates 1 unit*.

Again, diabetics in this country rarely need to be concerned about matching syringes to insulin strengths because U-100 is the only strength available here.

Virtually everyone today uses disposable syringes and needles that are made of plastic. These can be used a few times (as long as the needles are sharp) without too much concern about sterility. Be sure to recap the needle after each use and don't clean it with alcohol because it will remove the slick coating that lets it slide in easily. Dispose of it safely (see page 159) when it's dull or if it has touched anything but your own skin.

Today's smaller-gauge needles are slim, sharp, and specially coated to slide into the skin smoothly. The thinnest ½-inch needles—26, 27, 28, 29, 30, or 31 gauge—cause the least discomfort and are the most popular. Then there are the pediatric syringes that allow you to measure only ½ cc units. These syringes are great not only for small children but also for brittle diabetics who are extremely sensitive to insulin and may need adjustments in tiny doses.

The thinner the needle, the less discomfort it causes, so the 31-gauge is the least painful. It has one problem, however, and that is that it may not go in deep enough, so you'll have to see how it works on your own skin. Try them all out and decide which is best for you.

When you travel, take along a doctor's prescription for syringes and insulin plus a letter from the doctor stating that you are a diabetic. If you have problems away from home getting supplies, try a hospital emergency room.

ALLERGIC REACTIONS TO INSULIN

One problem that many insulin-dependent diabetics have always had is an allergic response at the site of the injection, especially when they have just started to take insulin or when they take it only occasionally. Often it occurs six or more weeks after starting to take injections. The symptoms—redness, swelling, itchiness—are usually mild and localized and completely gone in a couple of weeks.

Allergic reactions have become almost a problem of the past because they are seldom caused by the latest insulins, especially with "human insulin" that is made by gene-splicing. It may make us feel less than godlike to realize that the 51 amino acids of pig insulin differ only by one amino acid from the human. The cow, on the other hand, is three amino acids, plus some hoofs and a tail, away. The human insulins, made by neither pigs nor cows but bacteria or yeast, show no difference at all from the insulin made by the human body, although occasional allergic reactions have been reported.

HOW TO GIVE YOURSELF AN INJECTION

Though it seems very simple to an experienced person, injecting yourself is frightening for the beginner until you get the hang of it. Many people practice on something other than themselves—an orange, for example—until they have perfected a smooth technique. Even if you don't take insulin but control your diabetes with diet or oral agents, you must know how to inject it because a time may come—during an illness, perhaps—when you may require it temporarily. Ask your doctor to show you how to inject yourself and have all of the necessary supplies ready, just in case you need them in a hurry.

GETTING READY: THE MATERIALS YOU NEED
Here's what you will need at hand:

1. Insulin.
2. A disposable syringe that corresponds to the strength of your insulin. You merely unwrap it, use it, and dispose of it (or use it a few times before disposing of it).
3. Alcohol (70 percent ethyl/91 percent isopropyl).
4. Absorbent cotton or prepackaged alcohol swabs.

FILLING THE SYRINGE WITH INSULIN

1. Remember to keep the needle sterile. Don't touch it with your fingers or anything else.
2. Shake the insulin bottle gently, inverting it to make sure it is thoroughly mixed.
3. Wipe off the rubber stopper on the top of the bot-

tle with a piece of alcohol-soaked cotton. Do not remove the stopper from the bottle.

4. Draw the plunger back to the mark on the syringe
that corresponds with your dose of insulin. This fills the
space with air.

5. Insert the needle through the rubber stopper into
the bottle. Push the plunger all the way down, pushing
the air into the bottle.

6. With the needle in the bottle, turn the bottle upside
down and pull the plunger back *just beyond* the mark
showing your correct dose.

7. Slowly push the plunger back to the correct mark
for your dose. This will expel the air bubbles. Don't worry
about a few little bubbles. They won't hurt you. You
would require much more air than that to do you in.

8. When the syringe is filled with the correct dose, pull
the needle out of the bottle. Don't let the bottle hang upright on the needle because the needle may bend.

MIXING TWO INSULINS IN ONE SYRINGE

Let's suppose your doctor has instructed you to take 4
Regular and 10 NPH units of insulin.

1. Draw air into the syringe up to the 10-unit line.

2. Put the needle through the center of the rubber cap
of the NPH (cloudy) bottle and inject the 10 units of air
into the bottle.

3. Withdraw the needle, *empty.*

4. Draw 4 units of air into the same syringe.

5. Push the needle through the rubber cap of the Regular bottle (this insulin is clear) and inject this air into the
bottle.

6. Withdraw with 4 units of Regular insulin.

7. Turn the NPH bottle upside down and insert the
same needle into that bottle.

8. Slowly pull the plunger back to total 14 units. You now have 4 units of Regular and 10 units of NPH in your syringe.

NOTE: Regular must be injected immediately after mixing so it does not lose any of its strength. Regular mixed with NPH must also be injected immediately because, on standing, its composition can change.

Remember that Lantus or Levemir cannot be mixed with any other insulin in the same syringe.

INJECTING VERY FAST-ACTING INSULIN
The very fast-acting insulins—Humalog, NovoLog, and Apidra—may be injected anywhere in the body.

INJECTING REGULAR OR NPH
Using the older generations of insulin requires a little more planning because it does matter where they are injected. These insulins may be injected into the *fronts* of your thighs (the most commonly chosen site); the *backs* and *sides* of your upper arms; the *front* and *sides* of your abdomen; or the *top* of your buttocks. To be sure to avoid major blood vessels or nerves, never inject into the outsides of your thighs, the lower or inner areas of the buttocks, or below the knee. Be careful to stay far away from the radial nerve that is located near your elbow. Do not inject into scar tissue, which can't absorb the insulin. Because fatty tissue provides the best locations, a really thin person will usually use the thighs or buttocks, while fatter people have more options.

CHOOSING THE SPOT
It's always a good idea to rotate your sites so that you don't continually inject in the same spot, although this is not anywhere as important now that we are using bio-

logically identical human insulins. Remember that the rate of absorption varies in different parts of the body, so it is best to stick with the same anatomical area such as the thighs or the abdomen. If you don't compensate for the difference, you may throw your control off. When you inject in your abdomen, for example, the insulin is absorbed much more quickly than in your leg.

If you always inject yourself in the same spot, you could get a buildup of tissues called lipohypertrophy. Don't continue to inject yourself in these lumpy areas because it can delay the absorption of the insulin. Try to systematically change your injection site to avoid the problem.

If you want to inject your abdomen or arm, an area you probably do not usually use, you may have to reduce your dose by about 5 units unless your sugar is high and you want to take advantage of the greater absorption. If you aren't aware of the differences, you may have some unexpected reactions.

Just to confuse matters, it is important to remember that insulin absorption also increases if you inject in an area that is going to get immediate heavy exercise. So, if you are going to go biking, don't inject in your leg. If you'll be playing tennis, don't choose your racquet arm. Unless, of course, you have high sugar and want to bring it down in a hurry.

INJECTING THE INSULIN
Wipe the area with a piece of cotton soaked in alcohol, or a prepared alcohol swab. With one hand, pinch a large fold of flesh between your thumb and forefinger at least three inches apart. Or, to inject into your upper arm, lean against a door to push your flesh up.

With the other hand, pick up the syringe like a pencil or a dart. Push the needle quickly and firmly into the skin, straight in, perpendicular to the skin. (For small children and very thin people, a 45-degree angle may be better.) Pull back slightly on the plunger with the needle in place. If blood appears at the tip of the syringe, you have hit a small blood vessel. This isn't dangerous but may cause bleeding and bruising. (There's no harm in continuing with the injection, however, rather than withdrawing the needle.) Try to take no longer than about five seconds for the whole job. Now release the pinch and press an alcohol pad next to the needle and pull it out.

To prevent the possibility of a clogged needle, always inject the insulin *quickly* after pushing in the needle. But if the needle does clog, withdraw it and *write down* the number of units you have injected (your original dose minus the number of units remaining in the syringe). Take a new syringe and inject *only* the amount you still need to complete your full dose.

Occasionally you may notice that a little insulin squirts out when you make your injection and you don't know how many units you have lost. Or, as you take the needle out, there is more than the usual flow of blood, and again, you wonder if you have lost insulin. *Never* give yourself another injection. Probably you have not lost much, so simply eat a little less, and check your blood before lunch and dinner. If your sugar is high, you may need an extra dose (perhaps 4 to 5 units) of Regular insulin. Check with your doctor.

USING A PEN INJECTOR

If you hate to stick needles into yourself, even though they are so sharp and thin today that the prick is hardly noticeable, try a pen insulin injector. Insulin pens have become very popular not only for this reason but also because they are so convenient, especially for people who take multiple doses a day. In addition, they are handy for travelers. Lightweight and compact, they are small enough to fit in your pocket or handbag, so you don't have to carry syringes and bottles of insulin around with you.

Although most people like the pen injectors, some diabetics are more comfortable using syringes, especially after years of injections, because they can watch the insulin going in, something they can't do with a pen. But the pens are just as safe.

The pens combine an insulin container and a syringe and come in two varieties: reusable and prefilled. With the reusable pen, a cartridge containing 3 cc units of insulin is loaded into the pen and a needle is attached. Set the dose you want, press the pen against your skin, and push the button to trigger the disposable needle.

Each prefilled pen injector is loaded with 300 units of insulin and is discarded when finished.

A few precautions: As with any insulin, the prefilled pens or cartridges must not be frozen or exposed to very high temperatures. Unopened, they may be stored in the refrigerator and will be good until the expiration date, but the minute you take them out and take your first dose, they must not be returned to the refrigerator. Once they are opened, you should keep them at room temperature.

Depending on the kind of insulin they contain, the disposable pens and the cartridges are good for a specified length of time, ranging from 7 to 28 days, after they are opened. Be sure to check the labels.

Pens filled with Lantus insulin should be thrown away after a month, even if it's still half full. Levemir is good for about 42 days and then it, too, should be disposed of.

Do not use the insulin if it has been frozen or stored at high temperatures because its chemistry may have been altered. Do not use it after the expiration date on the label.

Before giving yourself a shot, shoot one or two units of insulin into the air to be sure the pen is working properly; then redial the dose.

Never carry a pen with a needle attached, unless its cover is on, because this leaves an open passageway for germs to get into the insulin.

It's best to change the needle every time you use it because it can become clogged or contaminated. Do not wash the needle with alcohol because you will remove the silicone coating that makes the injection easy and painless.

Always check the expiration date printed on the packaging before you buy pens or cartridges to make sure there's enough time for you to use the entire amount. No sense wasting your money. On the other hand, if you're using Lantus or Levemir in small doses, buy the 300-unit pen or cartridge so you won't have to waste a lot of it when you throw it away after a month or 42 days.

GUIDE TO PEN INSULINS

Humulin 70/30 Pen	Novolin Innolet 70/30
Humulin N Pen NPH	Novolin Innolet N Pen
Humalog Pen	NovoLog FlexPen
Humalog Mix 75/25 Pen	NovoLog Mix 70/30 FlexPen
Novolin 70/30 FlexPen	NovoPen 3

IF YOUR VISION IS POOR

If you can't see the numbers on the syringe, you may be glad to know that you can buy special inexpensive products that magnify the syringe and its numbers. Others enable you to tell with your fingers when you have filled the syringe with the prescribed dose of insulin. One device, for example, clicks as it counts off a certain number of units of insulin; another has gauges to measure units, while yet another measures a preset dose. Most of the devices are available from The Lighthouse (800-334-5497).

STORING YOUR INSULIN

Once you have opened a bottle of insulin or an injector, keep it in a cool, dim place, and be careful not to subject it to extreme temperatures.

Store your extra, *unopened* bottles or insulin cartridges in the refrigerator, but *never* put them in the freezer. Freezing destroys the insulin's potency. If a bottle freezes, throw it out. Never let it get very hot either. Don't keep it in your car's glove compartment, or on a windowsill in the sun or near the oven.

Insulin is marked with an expiration date. Check it before you buy it. After that date, even an unopened bottle may start losing its strength. In an emergency, outdated insulin may be used until you have a new supply. It loses strength very slowly. Under ordinary circumstances, though, if you see yours is outdated, don't use it.

The rules are different, however, for Lantus and Levemir, the newer very long-lasting insulins. As we have already said, once a bottle of Lantus has been opened, it should be thrown out after a month, even if it's still half full. Levemir is safe to use for 42 days after opening, but then it, too, must be tossed, whether or not you've used it up. If you're using a pen injector filled with Lantus or Levemir and you take small doses, better to use the 300-unit versions than those with larger doses because you won't waste so much of it.

Regular insulin must be clear and colorless, just like water. If it becomes cloudy or discolored, don't use it. The other insulins should not become granular or clumped. Insulin manufacturers have recently been saying that once a bottle has been used, you must discard it after a month, as it may lose some of its potency. I have not found this to be the case, but will go along with it.

INSULIN PUMPS

Insulin pumps have wrought near-miracles for many diabetics who have never before been able to achieve tight blood-sugar control. These people include many type 1 diabetics who are exceedingly hard to regulate, some type 2s who can't stay under control, some pregnant women, brittle diabetics who swing rapidly from one extreme of blood sugar to the other, and even some young children who otherwise face multiple injections a day. Most people can do very well without a pump, but occasionally it completely changes a poorly controlled diabetic's life.

Most insulin pumps are lightweight beeper-size, computerized, battery-powered devices that can be worn on your belt or carried in your pocket. They are programmed by you and your doctor to deliver a small trickle of short-acting insulin continuously around the clock, mimicking the normal release of insulin by the pancreas and keeping your blood glucose stable between meals and overnight. This is called basal or background insulin. If you require different basal amounts at different times of day, you can program the pump to provide those, too.

In addition to the basal insulin, the pump will also send a surge (bolus) of short-acting insulin when you give it a special command before meals and large snacks. The amount will vary according to how much carbohydrate you plan to eat, how much physical activity you'll be doing, or how high your blood sugar is at the moment. So you must check your blood sugar before every meal or snack.

Sounds complicated, and it is, but you'll be an expert in no time if you work at it.

THE INSULIN DISPENSER

One of the most recent varieties of the pump is a small lightweight insulin dispenser designed for type 2 diabetics who take insulin and want to avoid taking multiple injections a day. Quite tiny, this device is taped on your abdomen, arm, or leg and delivers 0.6 units of insulin continuously around the clock via a 31-gauge needle. This is your basal dose that never changes. To add your mealtime fast-acting insulin, you push a small button before you sit down to eat. The entire unit is discarded every 24 hours and replaced by another.

All this is done by way of an infusion set, a long thin tube with a needle or catheter at the end that is inserted under your skin in rotated sites, usually on the abdomen. Depending on your needs, the pump can hold a one- or two-day supply of insulin.

Although the pump should be worn day and night, it's possible to remove it for an hour or so for lovemaking, a bath, or a very special occasion.

The pump simulates as closely as possible the insulin output of a normal pancreas in response to food and has been responsible for impressive results for some diabetics who never imagined they could do so well.

On the other hand, the pump is not without problems. You can't just set it and forget it. It is awkward. It can cause infections at the infusion sites. The tubes can get clogged and the mechanism can fail, so it should be checked regularly. If you suspect trouble, call the 24-hour toll-free number found on the back of the device for technical advice. Meanwhile, test your blood glucose and inject your insulin yourself with a syringe or insulin pen, if necessary. Always keep such equipment handy in case you need it.

Pumps are expensive, and monthly maintenance can be high. They require careful training, supervision, and practice to use correctly. Blood sugar must be monitored at least four times a day.

If you are an orderly, organized, highly motivated, and perhaps compulsive person, the pump could be your answer. But for most people, if their numbers are good it is probably best to do without one.

PICK YOUR PUMP

Among the newer varieties of insulin pumps is a wireless combination system consisting of a glucose monitor and an "intelligent" insulin pump. The monitor sends blood sugar readings to a subcutaneous continuous insulin pump that takes the readings, along with other information contributed by you, and calculates the amount of insulin bolus needed. You then give it a command to deliver that amount. It is expected that this technology will soon lead to fully automated glucose monitoring and insulin-delivery systems that will deliver the appropriate doses.

Experts agree that while these pumps are not for everyone, they can definitely make life easier for just about all type 1 diabetics, as well as a minority of type 2s who can't seem to keep themselves under control despite multiple daily insulin injections. But having a pump doesn't mean you are home free. It's a lot of work, you still have to watch what you eat, and you have to monitor your blood glucose several times a day.

MULTIPLE INJECTIONS

To get optimum control, even more than two shots a day are required by some people. Obviously, if you can do well without multiple injections you won't want them, because this regime is not easy or fun. But it is well worth the bother if this is the only way you can maintain good control. Your gains are far greater than your efforts.

On the other hand, some compulsive patients insist on checking their blood sugar as often as five or six or seven times a day and taking insulin accordingly. This is not necessary. No need to become so obsessed by your diabetes that it's all you think about.

Of course, most insulin-taking diabetics must take multiple injections during stress periods, such as an illness or a pregnancy. And extremely variable or brittle diabetics often need them to cut down on severe reactions.

Whether you take the multiple injections on a daily basis or only temporarily, your insulin intake must be adjusted according to your test results. For example, when you take long-acting Lantus (glargine) or Levemir (detemir) at bedtime, you should start the morning off with a sugar level between 100 and 130 mgs. If you find that, instead, you are consistently falling in the 200 range before breakfast, you know you're not getting enough of the long-acting insulin and should increase it by a few units every few days until you reach the magic number. On the other hand, if you are consistently high before dinner every evening, you might need to give yourself a second smaller shot of Lantus or Levemir before breakfast to provide you with a more even blood-sugar level during the day.

To complicate your life, here's more advice. To determine whether you are taking enough very fast-acting insulin such as Humalog, NovoLog, or Apidra before each meal, for a couple of days check your blood again two hours after lunch, dinner, and bedtime to see if you're in the ballpark.

HELPING INSULIN WORK BETTER

A new drug called Symlin (pramlintide) is a synthetic injectable form of a natural hormone that provides additional help in regulating blood sugar and is prescribed for people who take very large doses of insulin but still find that they can't get their glucose down to an acceptable level.

This drug delays gastric emptying, counteracts a substance called amylin that works against the action of insulin, and helps in preserving the life span of the beta cells.

Symlin does, however, increase the likelihood of hypoglycemia, so you must be especially vigilant about monitoring your sugar and watching out for the early signs of an insulin reaction.

HOW TO DISPOSE OF USED SYRINGES AND NEEDLES

Never toss used syringes, needles, or lancets directly into the trash can because they are medical waste that has had contact with human blood. You can buy an inexpensive piece of equipment called a safe-clip that clips, catches, and contains the needles. Or place these "sharps" in an opaque puncture-proof hard plastic container with a tight-fitting screw top. Don't use glass because it can break. Never use aluminum cans because they can bend. Label the container "infectious sharps waste." Seal it with heavy-duty tape, and put it in the garbage—*never* in a recycling bin, because it could pose a danger to workers and/or cause problems in the recycling process.

Your community may have special laws about syringe and needle disposal, so check with your local sanitation or public health department.

Some communities have special disposal programs where you can drop off your needles at designated collection sites in local doctors' offices, health clinics, household hazardous waste centers, and fire or police departments. Some mail-back services will send you sturdy containers for used needles that you return for proper disposal. And some pharmacies and hospitals accept used syringes.

"OOPS! I'VE MADE A MISTAKE!"

It happens to everyone. You forget to take your insulin, you take too much, or get the amounts mixed up. Don't panic. Here is how to deal with your mistakes:

FORGETTING TO TAKE YOUR INSULIN

Suppose you get up in the morning, eat your breakfast, go to work or school and suddenly in the middle of the day you realize you didn't take your morning shot.

Now you must take more Regular (because you are behind in the insulin you need) and less longer-acting (because there is less time before your next morning shot).

Let's suppose you normally take 10 Regular and 30

Intermediate-acting in the morning. If it is now about 11 A.M., take your injection, using slightly less but close to your normal dose. If you don't realize your omission until 3:30 in the afternoon and you start having symptoms of high sugar, take 20 Regular and 20 Intermediate. You need quicker action (therefore the increased Regular) over a shorter time span (therefore the decreased Intermediate).

Suppose you are at work or school or far from home when you realize you haven't taken your insulin. Call a doctor in the area and arrange to go to the office for a shot. Or go to the emergency room at the local hospital, telling the admitting clerk you cannot sit around waiting but must be attended to quickly. A third possibility is to get the name and telephone number of a drugstore in the area and then ask your own doctor to call this pharmacy and prescribe a syringe and insulin for you.

TAKING A DOUBLE DOSE

Suppose you take your shot, have your breakfast, and give yourself another shot by mistake. Once in a while this won't hurt you if you eat enough to compensate for it—but don't make a habit of it. Meantime, have a field day. Have all those ice cream sodas, chocolate sundaes, coconut cakes you've been longing for. Space them out during the day and have a good snack before bed. Set your clock for 3 A.M. Get up and have another snack if your blood-sugar level is still low. The next morning, start your usual regime.

REVERSING YOUR SPLIT DOSES

A common error is to take what you normally take in the morning (the larger portion of your split dose) in the afternoon before dinner. In other words, suppose you normally take 10 fast-acting Regular and 30 Intermediate in the morning, and 4 fast-acting Regular and 10 Intermediate before dinner. Today you take your morning dose and then, before dinner, you unthinkingly take the same dose again, much more than you should at that hour. Again, eating is the answer. Eat more at dinner. Have a large bedtime snack and set your alarm clock for 3 A.M. Get up and check your blood-sugar level. If it is low, have some more goodies.

PREPARING FOR AN EMERGENCY

Always have a bottle of fast-acting insulin stored in your refrigerator, even if you don't use it ordinarily. It will keep almost indefinitely, though you should replace it when it becomes outdated. However, once it's opened, discard it after a month. Fast-acting insulin is always used when you need quick action.

INSULIN IN FOREIGN COUNTRIES

Insulin may be purchased all over the world and it is the same as you buy at home, whether or not it is made by an American manufacturer. Just be sure to buy the U-100 strength, or, if you cannot, also buy a syringe that corresponds to the strength you will be using (see Chapter 15). When you are traveling, be sure to take along a letter from your doctor stating that you are a diabetic who requires insulin and syringes. Carry it with you at all times.

ARE YOU A BRITTLE DIABETIC?

A brittle diabetic is insulin-dependent, has extreme lack of control, with blood sugar that swings widely and rapidly from one extreme to the other, and so is in constant danger of insulin reaction on the one hand and acidosis on the other.

If you are a true brittle diabetic, you must follow all the rules very rigidly, checking your blood four times a day so you always know exactly where your sugar level stands. You should have a home glucose monitor (see the next chapter) so you can read your blood sugar in an instant. You may also be a candidate for an insulin pump.

Why you are unstable is a mystery in most cases, but some people are extremely sensitive to a difference of one or two units of insulin. Others, because of neuropathy, have stomachs that do not empty quickly and so glucose does not get into the bloodstream fast enough. Some have defects in their compensation mechanisms so the liver doesn't release sugar when it is needed. And perhaps there are other reasons we don't yet know about.

But, in most instances, brittle diabetics are not *really* brittle. They have simply never learned how to cope correctly with their condition. Perhaps their doctors have prescribed doses of insulin that are much too high. Then they eat too much to prevent reactions, thus raising their blood sugar way up, then take more insulin to bring it down, in a never-ending cycle. Perhaps they are not eating the correct diet, or have not tried taking insulin in split or multiple doses.

Or they may not know how to handle sick days, exercise days, or days of little activity.

Before you accept a diagnosis of "brittle," be sure you and your doctor have explored all the possibilities.

7

TESTING YOUR BLOOD SUGAR

Although there are many more enjoyable experiences in life, you must consistently test your blood for its sugar level. Testing is a diabetic's best friend because it tells you how well your body is handling the sugar it both produces internally and processes from the food you eat. It is a simple and essential procedure. You don't have to love it, but you have to do it.

All diabetics—whether their diabetes is controlled by diet alone, oral agents, or insulin—must test every day, sometimes multiple times a day, no matter how they feel.

Many diabetics insist they can *tell* when their sugar isn't normal. That's why they don't bother to make tests very often. If they feel "off," then they make a test. But the truth is, few people can detect sugar fluctuations unless those levels fall very low or rise very high. It is a rare person who will notice any true symptoms unless blood sugar is below 40 mgs or above 400, and some people don't notice them until their sugar goes much higher than that.

Find out for yourself. Note down your feelings, decide whether you feel normal, high or low, then test your blood four times a day for a couple of weeks. Were you always correct? It is extremely doubtful that you were.

WHY MUST YOU DO IT?

Why is testing important? Why, if you feel well, must you know your blood-sugar level? Because the effects of diabetes are cumulative, and it is well known today that consistently high or even moderately high sugar over a long period of time can help to bring about dire physical complications. It is very important that your sugar is consistently normal most of the time because high levels of blood sugar have an eventual deleterious effect on every organ of the body. You must also maintain a log of the test results so that glucose values can be tracked over time. Some glucose-testing monitors can be helpful because they have "memory" and will tell you when you last tested yourself. One even gives you the time of day the tests were taken.

HOW OFTEN SHOULD TESTS BE MADE?

You must test your sugar level at least once a day, whether you take medication or not. And you should keep a record of the results.

Diabetics who are controlled by diet alone and whose sugars are usually low can probably get along well with blood tests only once a day or even just a few times a week. The results will tell you whether your diet requires adjustment or whether you may require medication to keep your diabetes under control.

If you take oral hypoglycemic agents, a schedule of two tests a day—before breakfast and before dinner—will inform you about your control. If you are not doing well, then you must also test before lunch and bedtime until you see normal results once more. You must also adjust your diet so that the oral agents will be sufficient to help you produce or utilize enough of your own insulin to compensate for what you eat. If you cannot do that, you may have to increase your dose, switch to another kind of oral medication, or graduate to insulin injections.

If you take insulin, then tests must be made at least three times a day—before breakfast, dinner, and bedtime. In times of stress or illness, add a fourth test, before lunch. There's rarely a need to do it more often than that.

Each test gives you a report on the action of your medication vs. your food consumption and exercise during the immediately preceding period of time.

No matter what kind of diabetic you are, you must make at least four tests a day if you:

Have an infection, even a cold.

Feel nauseated or weak or have diarrhea.

Lose weight.

Are very thirsty or urinate more frequently than usual.

See any unusual pattern to your test results.

KEEP RECORDS

Isolated test results won't tell you or your doctor very much, except that *at this moment* your blood sugar is high or low. But if you write down the results after each test, you will be able to detect a pattern to your blood-sugar levels and can then correct for any aberrations. An isolated high or low result isn't very important, but consistent highs or lows will tell you and the doctor that a change must be made. Your diet, your medication, or your activity may require adjustments, or an undiagnosed illness may need treatment.

Write your test results in a notebook, and make short notations about how you feel, whether you are ill, tired, stressed, if you have overindulged in food, underindulged in exercise, had a bad night's sleep, suffered an emotional high or low, etc.

Read over your accumulated test results once or twice a week to see if there are any recurring patterns of abnormal readings of high or low sugar levels, so you can make your own adjustments or discuss your situation with your doctor. Take your records with you to the doctor.

IF YOU ARE SICK

Make tests at least four times a day, and test for acetone if your sugar is high. Talk to your doctor *at least once a day* for instructions about medication based on that day's test results (see Chapter 11).

TESTING FOR ACETONE

Whenever you get a sugar reading over 250 mgs twice in a row, it is imperative to test for the presence of acetones (or ketones) because, if you are producing these acids as a result of burning fat instead of carbohydrate, you *must* know it and correct it promptly. If you don't, you are setting forth on a short road to acidosis and plenty of trouble, so always keep test strips handy in case you need them and make sure they are not outdated. This advice applies to diabetics on oral agents as well as those on insulin because they too can get in trouble when they are sick.

If your urine reveals the presence of acetone as well as high sugar, *check with your doctor without delay* about what to do. Perhaps you'll be told to take more medication immediately or wait to see if the acetone decreases.

Test for it every two to four hours until it is completely gone. See Chapter 9 for more details.

When you test your urine for acetone, use Ketostix, Acetest, Chemstrip K, or a similar product, little plastic strips that contain two test areas, one for sugar and the other for acetone. Dip the strip in the urine. Wait 15 seconds, then compare the acetone square with the chart. If you have acetone, the square will turn lavender or purple.

Color	Amount of Acetone
No change	None
Lavender	Small amount
Light purple	Moderate amount
Dark purple	Large amount

If your blood test indicates that your blood sugar is low or normal although your acetone is high, that means you are not consuming enough carbohydrate. Nothing to worry about. Just correct your eating habits.

But, if your sugar is *high* and your acetone is *also high,* that's serious. *Call your doctor* because you will require more insulin than usual.

TESTING YOUR BLOOD SUGAR

Blood testing, which has almost totally replaced urine testing, gives you very specific blood-sugar readings. It tells you where you are *right now,* eliminating the time lag that is inevitable with urine testing.

Some mild well-controlled type 2 diabetics can get away with testing their blood only once a day or sometimes even less frequently. But for most people, at least a few times a week is highly recommended, and multiple tests every single day are essential for many others. They are especially essential if you are sick, if you are a type 1 diabetic who finds it hard to maintain control, a brittle diabetic who needs constant insulin adjustment, or if you are pregnant.

They are also useful to people who want to check the effect of certain foods on their blood sugars. For example, if you wonder if a scoop of ice cream, or an apple, or crackers will raise your blood sugar far out of bounds, check your sugar two hours after you have eaten them. If your blood is not abnormally elevated, you are home free.

Because there's no sense taking a blood-glucose test unless you are prepared to respond to the information it gives you, you must know how to adjust your medication, food, and exercise accordingly. This takes study, experience, and motivation, after a thorough discussion with your doctor.

HOW TO PRICK YOURSELF

It's astonishing—or maybe it isn't—how many people are afraid to prick themselves to get the necessary drop of blood for testing. But after you have done it a few times, you will see it isn't really traumatic. Besides, help is here for those of faint heart. In place of a lancet, today most people use automatic prickers. These spring-loaded devices release a lancet and need only to be pressed against your finger or another site to prick it automatically. Most people say this is almost painless.

Now, to get that drop of blood: Swab your finger with alcohol and let it dry. Press your thumb just under the tip of the finger to be used until the fingertip turns red. Make a small prick and squeeze out a large drop of blood. Drop the blood onto your test strip.

You can prick any part of your fingertips, but you will feel it least if you use the sides of the finger pads, because there are fewer nerve endings there. The thumb and the fourth finger are the least sensitive.

If you hate to prick your fingers, take heart. Results from a recent study show that drawing blood from the edge of your palm or heel of your hand is just as good as fingertip testing. The palm has plenty of blood capillaries and fewer pain receptors than the fingers and doesn't require buying a new glucose meter. You can also take blood from other parts of your body, such as your thigh, using a lancing device such as Vaculance or Freestyle.

TESTING THE OLD-FASHIONED WAY

Now, to see how much glucose is circulating in your bloodstream at this very moment, you may choose to use chemically treated test strips. Keep in mind that this method gives you only a rough indication of your sugar level, nowhere near as accurate as the readings you get with a blood-glucose meter. That's why this method is rarely used anymore. But here's how to do it.

Draw a drop of blood and place it on a strip. Wait 60 seconds, wipe the blood off with dry cotton, wait another 60 seconds. Compare the color with the guide on the container.

If the reading is more than 240 mgs percent, wait one more minute. It may move higher.

Even if you usually measure your blood glucose with a reflectance meter, you should know how to use these simple strips in case your machine malfunctions and you haven't been able to reach the manufacturer for technical advice. Better yet, have a second meter in reserve. They are not expensive.

USING A BLOOD-GLUCOSE MONITOR

For much more accurate readings of your blood sugar than you can get with the old-fashioned test strips, use an electronic home blood-glucose monitor that provides a snapshot of your sugar situation at that particular moment in time. Small enough to fit in your pocket, the meters are very simple to use. You touch the blood onto a small test strip that has been inserted into the monitor. It emerges in a few seconds with a digital readout of your blood-glucose level. Some of the newer machines eliminate one step in this process by including replaceable drums of strips that automatically eject the strips as they are used.

There are so many varieties of monitors available today, with more coming along every year, that you should discuss their merits with your physician before you make a choice. You should also check out the recommendations of the American Diabetes Association. Some meters are easier to use than others or perform tasks that the others don't, such as storing and recalling your last ten to fifty results. Some are more portable or more readable, and some have spoken instructions for the visually impaired. Others feature software kits that retrieve information from the meter and display past test results.

Among the newer, more sophisticated models is the MiniMed's Guardian Real Time, approved by the FDA in 2005. This one has a sensor inserted under the skin of the abdomen and a monitor that reads your blood-sugar level every five minutes from a distance of up to six feet. An alarm sounds when your sugar goes too high or too low, making it an excellent choice for people who are afraid to go to sleep at night for fear of having an insulin reaction during the night.

A real breakthrough is the Minimed Paradigm REAL-time System, also FDA-approved, the first combination glucose-monitor system and insulin pump. The monitor taped to your abdomen continuously reads your blood sugar and transmits the data to a pump that beeps when blood sugar drops to a dangerous level. Then the pump can be adjusted to administer additional insulin. This device gives you the closest thing yet to an artificial pancreas.

The FreeStyle Navigator by Abbott, currently being evaluated by the FDA, measures your sugar level through a patch worn on the skin and gives readings on a hand-held meter as often as every 60 seconds.

DexCom STS, already approved, is a short-term sensor worn on the body that transmits data wirelessly to a handheld receiver, making it comfortable to wear.

The long-heralded GlucoWatch or Glucoband that's meant to be worn on the wrist like a wristwatch and measures glucose levels through the skin is still in study.

And you may have heard about the meter that does not require blood but uses an infrared ray against the skin. A great idea but, because of development problems, it is still many years away.

Be sure to get detailed directions on how to use your monitor and then remember to follow them carefully. Test it at least once a month according to the manufacturer's instructions; recalibrate it when you open a new package of strips; don't use strips that are outdated or have changed color; keep the meter scrupulously clean; check its accuracy periodically by comparing its readings with your doctor's findings; wash your hands before using.

Prices for monitors vary widely. Most of them are very expensive, especially when you add the cost of the strips and the sensors that must be changed regularly and may not be covered by your health insurance. Check with your insurance company about reimbursement for everything you need.

Be aware that the meters may not always be accurate at very high altitudes or in extreme temperatures. Anemia, too, may affect their readings.

Some meters now allow you to test sites other than your fingertips. One model lets you take blood from the base of your thumb, palm, thigh, or even forearm, all of which are less painful than pricking your finger. A recent study, however, found that measurements with forearm blood weren't as accurate as those from finger sticks.

HbA1c: THE TEST THAT TELLS ALL

The blood-sugar tests we have been discussing give you important information about how good your control is today. The hemoglobin A1c test (HbA1c), a blood-sugar test made in a laboratory that requires a visit to your doctor, tells how you have been doing for the last two or three months. *It's the best way we have of knowing whether your sugar is under control and it should be done regularly in addition to your regular home monitoring.*

Because the hemoglobin A1c test tattles on you, reporting your past performance, it is especially important if you don't test often enough and tend to let your control slide. Or if you are one of those people who behave themselves for a week or so before each visit to the doctor but neglect their diabetes in between. Even though you know that consistently high sugars will cause disaster eventually, you may pay little attention until you get into trouble. This test, if it is made regularly, helps keep you on the path to righteousness.

Hemoglobin A1c is hemoglobin with glucose attached

to it. Normally it is only a tiny part of your total hemoglobin supply. But when you have elevated blood sugar, the glucose tends to stick to the hemoglobin A that makes up 97.5 percent of your red blood cells. The more sugar in your blood, the more saturated the hemoglobin A becomes. Once the cells have glucose attached to them, the sugar remains there throughout their lifespan—about 120 days.

By measuring the A1c, your doctor will know your overall blood-sugar level for the last couple of months. The normal range has long been considered to be somewhere between 3.2 and 6.2 percent, the equivalent of a blood-sugar level of 60 to 120 mgs, depending on the method used by the laboratory. However, the most recent research indicates that a maximum of 5.3 percent is what you should shoot for because its equivalent is a fasting blood-sugar level of 100 mgs. Keeping your HbA1c low definitely helps you avoid diabetic complications later on in life, so a high number indicates the need for prompt reform.

This test does not require fasting or repeated sampling, nor need it be done at any special time of day. It would be wise to have it made about every three months if you take oral agents or insulin. Meantime, don't forget your daily home tests. Getting optimal A1c levels requires daily blood-glucose measurements of 90 to 130 before meals, or less than 180 after a meal.

Occasionally, the hemoglobin A1c test fails to give accurate or useful results. The reason could be that it hasn't been made within the correct time limits or at a reliable laboratory; or the results could be skewed by wide swings in your blood-sugar levels just before undergoing the test. However, in almost all cases it is an excellent indication of your control during the last couple of months. A 1 percent drop in your A1c score greatly reduces your risk of developing diabetic complications. For example, it will cut your risk of nerve damage, vision loss, and kidney disease by about a third.

By the way, there are kits for measuring A1c at home, but we don't recommend them. It is much safer to have the test done at your doctor's office when you go for your checkups every three months.

FRUCTOSAMINE TEST: ANOTHER TATTLETALE

If you—and your doctor—don't want to wait three months between tests to find out if you've been keeping your blood sugars under good control, a fructosamine test is another way to keep you honest. This measures the amount of glucose that attaches not to hemoglobin but to a different substance in the blood. Unlike the A1c test, which measures your blood glucose over the last two or three months, the fructosamine test issues a report on your control over the preceding two weeks. It is useful when you're making a change in your regime because you can tell right away whether your sugars are improving. It's useful for your doctor who may suspect you've not been faithful to your diet.

8

INSULIN REACTIONS

When you are an insulin-taking diabetic, you quickly learn that you have a major concern which hardly anybody else ever worries about or knows exists. That's insulin reaction, very low blood sugar (hypoglycemia) caused by the presence of too much insulin in your bloodstream. Unless you are always spilling sugar (a bad idea), it is inevitable that you will have an occasional reaction, usually minor and easily handled. While reactions can hardly be described as delightful experiences, they are far healthier than having consistently high blood sugar, which in time can do inexorable damage to your body.

Besides, reactions can usually be avoided, and certainly minimized, by using your common sense.

In the nondiabetic, insulin is produced by the islet cells of the pancreas in response to the level of sugar in the bloodstream. The amount is always just enough to cover the sugar, and there is never too much. If the blood-glucose level falls too low, the liver releases more sugar from its standby stores, again just the right amount to do the job.

But diabetics who require exogenous insulin do not run on automatic. They must try to match the amount of insulin they take with the blood sugar they *expect* to have. Sometimes, for various reasons, they have too much insulin in their bloodstream, and the blood-sugar level falls too low. When this happens, the brain and the central nervous system do not have the glucose they need for fuel and start to function less efficiently. The result is an insulin reaction.

DIET ALONE OR ORAL AGENTS

If you are a diabetic who is treated with diet alone, you will *never* have insulin reactions. If you take oral agents, there is a remote possibility of reactions under certain circumstances, especially with the sulfonylureas, but I have seen only a few in all my years of practice. They occur in most cases only when there is a change in liver or kidney function, when overlapping medication is taken, or when the diabetic is elderly and frail, or is seriously ill and eats so poorly that he does not have an adequate store of glycogen ready to be released from the liver in emergencies. They can, however, be more severe than reactions from insulin, so take them seriously and report them to your doctor. One patient taking a sulfonylurea was given an antidepressant and had a reaction that lasted for almost a week.

Reactions can be severe because the sulfonylureas, unlike insulin that is quickly used up, stay in the system for days, perhaps causing the hypoglycemia to continue for days. The treatment is IV glucose given continuously until your sugar comes back up to normal.

WARNINGS AND SYMPTOMS

For an insulin-dependent diabetic, the possibility of a reaction begins when blood sugar falls below 40 or 50 mgs percent. Or when sugar takes a sudden nosedive, even if it goes from 400 to 200 mgs percent. The exact level as well as the symptoms vary for everyone.

Early warnings that a reaction is happening may include one or more of these feelings: weakness, sweating, headache, "butterflies" in the stomach, nausea, sudden hunger, anxiety, confusion, clumsiness, shakiness, pallor, palpitations, tingling of the lips, dizziness, a change in attitude, such as inappropriate laughing or crying. Also rapid heart rate, sweating, and apprehension. As someone has once described it, it's as if you have almost been hit by a train. Some people, on the other hand, feel very drowsy and may have an irresistible urge to yawn, while others find that their vision becomes blurred.

Still others get uncharacteristically hostile and irritable, angry, combative, and maybe even abusive. If the latter is true of you, don't worry. Your personality hasn't changed permanently, and with a little sugar you'll be right back to your old self.

These symptoms are all associated with a low supply of glucose to the brain, which needs sugar to function, plus the adrenaline your body releases into the bloodstream in an effort to raise your blood sugar.

Sometimes a headache is the only sign. Sometimes the feeling of being very tired for no particular reason is the sole warning signal. When this happens, don't go to sleep without checking to see if your blood sugar is low. If it is, you are probably starting to have a reaction.

If the reaction is allowed to continue, the symptoms may progress to slurred speech, mental confusion, dilated pupils, instability, and eventually to convulsions and loss of consciousness. A good rule for all insulin-taking diabetics: Before driving, count backward from 100 by sevens. If you can't do it, test your blood and, if necessary, take sugar immediately.

WHAT CAUSES REACTIONS?

The low blood sugar that leads to a reaction is caused by just three things:

Taking too much insulin (sometimes by mistake).
Not eating when and what you should.
Exercising more than usual without compensating with
   extra calories or less insulin.

Reactions usually happen just before a meal, or when your insulin has its peak effect (see Chapter 6). With the very long-acting insulins such as Lantus (glargine) and Levemir (detemir) that don't have major peaks, you won't have to be so concerned about reactions.

THE GOOD NEWS ABOUT REACTIONS

Insulin reactions are no fun, but even if you go through a severe episode, complete with unconsciousness and perhaps amnesia, they won't kill you. Nor will they cause brain damage. Think of all the children who have had multiple insulin reactions and have gone on to get Ph.Ds. Reactions can, however, be most inconvenient and embarrassing for you and, at the same time, frightening to the people around you, especially the uninitiated who may have no idea what's wrong or how to help you.

PREVENTION IS COMMON SENSE

If you know what triggers reactions, then you can almost always avoid them or head them off quickly.

• Always eat *on time* and eat *enough*. Never skip a meal unless you take less insulin. Don't forget your scheduled snacks.

• Be extremely careful when you measure out your insulin, double-checking to be sure you are taking the correct dose.

• If you are going to do more exercise than usual, eat more carbohydrate in preparation for it, or take less insulin, or both (see Chapter 4). Consult with your doctor to determine amounts. Before you set out to exercise, always test your blood for sugar. If it is low before you even begin, then you surely need to make adjustments.

Look out for reactions the day *after* heavy exercise, when your liver may still be depleted of its supply of extra glycogen. So if you run the marathon or spend all day Sunday giving the house a thorough spring cleaning, watch your step on Monday. Be sure to test your blood sugar. Your food, which normally would go into blood sugar, is now funneled into your liver to be stored, so you may need more food (or less insulin) on Monday in order to prevent hypoglycemia.

During your exercise, especially if it is strenuous and prolonged, it is quite possible you need some additional sugar. (Most people don't think of sex as exercise, but it is. Eat a snack before jumping into bed.)

• Anytime you'll be driving for more than a half hour—especially after exercise or a long day at work—check your blood sugar *before* you get in the car. If it is low or on the verge of low, *eat something*. Always have some form of sugar handy, in your pocket and in the glove compartment, ready to use. If it is *high*, however, do *not* take extra insulin, not even a few units. Wait until you are home to make a correction.

• Sometimes, perhaps on a Saturday or Sunday, you may sleep late and skip breakfast. Since you are only going to eat two meals that day, be sure to take less insulin.

• An occasional reaction is nothing to be concerned about, but if yours happen frequently, then you are doing something wrong. Usually the answer is that your insulin dosage is too high, or you are not eating enough at the right times. Review your diet and make sure you are eating a consistent number of calories that include the correct amount of carbohydrates. Check out your snacks. Are you getting enough carbohydrate and protein? There is *always* a reason for frequent reactions and you must find it.

Sometimes reactions tend to occur at the same time of day or night. Then you will know, *if you are eating correctly,* that your dose must be reevaluated and adjusted. Too much fast-acting Regular insulin taken in the morning often causes reactions before lunch. Too much NPH may precipitate afternoon reactions when its action peaks. Your dose may be too high. Or you may do better with split amounts, giving you smaller but more frequent doses. Or switch to Lantus or Levemir, which do not peak and therefore don't usually cause such problems.

Let your doctor know about your reactions and request that you review your dose, your diet, and your exercise together. If you continue to have problems, perhaps you should go to another doctor, one whose specialty is diabetes.

OTHER POSSIBILITIES

• The rate of absorption of the insulin you inject is affected by *where* you inject it. We know that the abdomen and arms usually have higher and faster absorption rates than the legs. If your reactions tend to occur after you have used these sites, maybe this is the reason. You can use this information to your advantage, not only to explain and prevent reactions but to help you overcome high sugars more rapidly. When your sugar is high, injecting in your abdomen or arm can bring it down more rapidly.

• Pregnancy has a tremendous effect on your insulin needs (see Chapter 13), and you will probably require much less insulin in the first trimester (first 13 weeks) when the fetus and the placenta consume a lot of your circulating sugar and when you may not be eating as much as you usually do. This is a time when reactions are very common and can be severe. During the rest of your pregnancy, you will undoubtedly require much *more* insulin than usual. But after the baby is born, your insulin needs will drop again—another time when you must be especially alert to the possibility of insulin reactions.

• The insulin requirements of menstruating women can be variable, too. Some women find it hard to keep their blood sugar on target during their menstrual cycles, usually the week *before* their periods but sometimes during them. Keep track of the pattern of your blood sugar at those times and discuss it with your doctor and your gynecologist.

• Your emotional state can affect your need for more or less insulin. Although chronic stress seems to raise blood sugar, acute stress can lower it in a hurry, causing a reaction.

• Vomiting or diarrhea may deplete your body of the sugar it needs to function. You must get sugar somehow to avoid a reaction, so if you can't eat, drink regular (not diet) ginger ale for nourishment, take an antiemetic, such as Compazine or Tigan in suppository form or by injection. And *immediately* call your doctor. You may need intravenous glucose if nothing else does the job (see Chapter 11). Be aware that one out of about 500 people gets an adverse reaction to Compazine.

• Too much alcohol consumption, too, can be the reason for insulin reactions because it inhibits the release of glucose from the liver when you need it. Not only that, it may make you forget to eat on time.

• Certain drugs can have an effect on your insulin requirements. For example, beta blockers such as Inderal, Lopressor, or Tenormin, prescribed for hypertension, can mask the reactions so you won't be aware you're about to have one and you won't realize you need food.

• Some people, especially those who have had diabetes for many years, have "hypoglycemia unawareness." In other words, they don't experience the usual warning signs heralding the onset of low blood sugar before lapsing into a full-fledged insulin reaction. If you are among those who don't always know when their glucose level is dropping, be sure to cover yourself by testing your blood frequently.

• A caution for sauna devotees: A study has found that a sauna following your insulin injection can increase the absorption rate by 110 percent. So, have your sauna *after* a meal or snack, take along some carbohydrate, and since you won't be wearing your clothes or carrying your wallet card, be sure to wear your ID bracelet or necklace.

• Reactions can cause blurred vision, dizziness, and fuzzy thinking, so take special care when you're driving or operating machinery. Be sure your blood sugar isn't too low before you start, and have a snack every half hour or so if you stay at it for a long time. Remember the suggestion of counting backward from 100 by sevens.

• Hot or very cold weather also seems to affect some

people's sugar metabolism because more energy is expended, especially when the extreme temperatures are combined with exercise. Be on the alert for reactions.

NIGHTTIME REACTIONS

Many people, especially before their insulin dosage is adjusted properly, have reactions during the night or in the early morning. If this is the case with you, you should always, without fail, remember to eat a snack before bedtime. If there is no reason to suspect the hypoglycemia is caused by more exercise than usual that day or less food than you normally consume, *then your answer lies in your insulin dose.* You are taking too much Intermediate- or long-acting insulin in the morning. The doctor may suggest decreasing it by about 4 units to see if the nighttime reactions stop. If your daytime sugars go higher as a result, then a small amount of Regular insulin can be added to the syringe in the morning. Make changes in your dose only after consulting your doctor.

REACTIONS WITHOUT WARNING

You may be one of those diabetics who, after having had the disease for many years, tend to get reactions without any warning at all. If so, you must try even harder to avoid them. Test your blood four times a day. Be sure to have snacks at 10:30 A.M., 3:30 P.M., and before you go to bed, whether or not you think you need them. Include in your bedtime snack some protein (i.e., cheese or milk) as well as carbohydrate. During the night, your body will slowly convert that protein to usable carbohydrate.

KNOW YOUR BLOOD SUGAR

Diabetics who take insulin must test their blood a few times a day. If you keep a record of your sugars, you will be able to tell if there is a pattern to your episodes of hypoglycemia. You'll know if they seem to be caused by specific happenings in your life. You will also know when you must eat more or take less insulin so you won't have reactions.

When you know exactly where your blood sugar stands at any given moment, you can start to plan small adjustments in your eating or insulin schedules as needed.

REACT TO A REACTION *FAST*

If you suspect you are beginning to have a reaction, don't wait around to see what's going to happen. Don't fight it. Do something right *now*. You may not have much time before you are in real trouble. Even if you are not sure that what you feel is a reaction, even if you think perhaps these symptoms may be caused by high sugar rather than low and you don't have the time or the facilities to test your blood sugar immediately, take preventive measures at once. In this case, better safe than sorry really applies.

Treatment at this stage is easy. Eat something. If the reaction is mild, some carbohydrate and protein (perhaps a glass of milk and some crackers) is sufficient. If it seems more pronounced or you tend to have reactions that come upon you quickly, take rapidly absorbed sugar: 2 teaspoons of granulated sugar—plain or dissolved in a little water (pilfer a few of those little packets of sugar the next time you're in a restaurant); a small tube of confectioner's sugar; 6 or 7 Lifesavers or hard candies; 4 ounces of orange or apple juice or regular (not diet) soft drink; 2 teaspoons of honey or corn syrup; a handful of raisins; whatever is handy and appeals to you most.

Some diabetics carry sugar cubes, glucose tablets (these come in packs of three and are easy to carry around with you), or little tubes of "Instant Glucose" with them. This is 25 grams of concentrated sugar that can be squeezed right into your mouth and absorbs very quickly. Or tubes of cake icing straight from the grocery store.

Don't overshoot the mark and take so much sugar that you will pay for it later in high blood sugar. You need 10 or 15 or, at most, 20 grams of sugar. After you have taken the sugar, *wait*. It takes 10 or 15 minutes for it to be absorbed into the bloodstream and reach your brain. If you don't start to feel better after 15 minutes, eat more.

Some people are so frightened of reactions that they start eating and keep on eating until the feelings have passed. By then they have so overdosed that it takes them days to get their blood sugar down to normal again. It is like killing a fly with a .22 rifle.

When you have recovered from your reaction, remember that you've given yourself a quick fix by ingesting pure sugar. It helps temporarily until the sugar is sopped up by the liver and muscles that need to restore their depleted supplies. Now you are low on blood sugar again and you could have another reaction. You need some protein, perhaps a glass of milk with two crackers, a scoop of ice cream, or peanut butter, all of which will convert slowly into carbohydrate.

Obviously, the fuel you may need in a hurry must always be readily available to you. Carry some supplies in your pocket or handbag at all times, in the car's glove compartment, your suitcase, the desk drawer. One man keeps his in the top of his sock when he runs; another ties a little bag of sugar packets to his belt. No matter where you stash it, your emergency supplies must literally be at hand.

Important: Make a frequent check on your cache of sweets. Somebody else may have eaten them. Or perhaps you used them and forgot to stock up again.

BACK TO YOUR NORMAL SCHEDULE

After you have taken extra food in response to a reaction, do not cut back on your regular eating plan. Forget you had it and eat as usual. That sugar is not to be calculated as part of your daily diet.

Your blood sugar will rebound within about an hour after treating a reaction with sugar, sometimes going as high as 200 or 300 mgs. Don't take extra insulin to counteract it, but test your blood again before your next meal.

WHAT OTHER PEOPLE SHOULD KNOW

Just in case you'll ever have a severe reaction and can't respond to it yourself, train your family, responsible friends, and colleagues to know what to do. If you are in school, your teachers should know. Tell them that if you are conscious, they should give you the quickly absorbed sweets described on page 185, even if you object. Your low sugar when you have a reaction may make you stubborn!

A good trick for them to use if you refuse to open your mouth is to hold your nose closed so that you have to open your mouth to breathe. Of course, orange juice usually does the job, but it can be messy if you are not cooperative. Those little tubes of glucose that look like toothpaste tend to work better. If the glucose is squeezed into your mouth, you'll have to swallow it, and in short order you'll be in a position to take food on your own.

If you are unconscious, that is another story. Nothing should be forced into your mouth because you may aspirate it, compounding your problems. Now you will require intravenous glucose or an injection of glucagon, a hormone produced by the pancreas that raises blood sugar in a hurry. That may mean someone will have to call 911 so EMS can do it for you. But the call can probably be avoided if you are prepared with a glucagon emergency kit.

KEEP A KIT HANDY

You would be wise to keep a glucagon emergency kit handy and make sure the people around you know how to use it, especially if you are prone to sudden and severe reactions. It requires a prescription and is available at drugstores. The kit, complete with instructions, consists of a vial of liquid and a vial of powder that are mixed together and then injected anywhere in your body. Just about anybody could do it for you.

It is extremely rare that one injection does not solve the problem of extreme hypoglycemia. It will probably bring you around in about 10 minutes and then you can take sugar by mouth. But if you don't respond, a second shot will not be effective. You must be seen by a doctor immediately or taken to a hospital emergency room for intravenous glucose infusion or other treatment.

Be sure someone in your family and at school or work

knows how to give glucagon injections. It is very simple and requires no medical knowledge or expertise.

By the way, if you have a hypoglycemic reaction as the result of an overdose of alcohol, the glucagon kit may not do the trick. Alcohol inhibits the conversion of protein to carbohydrate and lowers the sugar level even more. So if you've gone on a real toot (we're not talking here about casual drinking, which usually means two drinks for a man, one for a woman) and have a severe response, be sure your drinking companions know to call EMS *immediately*. By the way, you *should* know that wine and beer consumed in enough quantity will affect you as much as hard liquor.

THE DIFFERENCE BETWEEN INSULIN REACTION AND ACIDOSIS

Because acidosis, which we will discuss in the next chapter, can also lead to coma, it is sometimes difficult for you or another layperson to know the difference when you begin to feel peculiar or actually pass out. When in doubt, however, treat yourself for a reaction if you haven't the time to take a test, because insulin shock can lay you out very quickly. Diabetic coma happens gradually.

The best indication of an insulin reaction is profuse sweating, as opposed to acidosis, when you hardly sweat at all. In acidosis, even your tongue and your armpits, a heavy source of sweat glands, will be dry because you have lost so much water in excessive urination.

Of course, the best way to know whether your sugar is low or high is to make a quick blood test, if you have time.

LABEL YOURSELF

Not only should you let everyone with whom you associate know you are a diabetic who may have reactions, but it is most important to wear or carry something that identifies you as a diabetic—a bracelet, a necklace, and/or a wallet card that explains who you are and what to do in emergencies. It will let people know how to act in an emergency, and will help keep you out of the local jail, where many diabetics land when their behavior or lack of consciousness is misinterpreted as overindulgence in alcoholic spirits.

As a precaution, carry identification with you that says you are a diabetic and explains what should be done for you in an emergency. A simple way to do this is to join MedicAlert (800–344–3226 or www.medicalert.com). For a small fee, you get a wallet card and a stainless-steel bracelet or neck chain engraved with your personal identification number, and a 24-hour-a-day toll-free telephone number. Information about your treatment is kept on file and is available to you or medical personnel who may need it in an emergency. Included in the file are the names and telephone numbers of your physician and people to notify in an emergency and other relevant material.

9

COPING WITH ACIDOSIS

Though the rights to insulin reactions belong almost entirely to diabetics who take insulin, this is not the case with acidosis or ketosis, at the other end of the blood-sugar spectrum. *No matter what kind of diabetic you are and whether or not you take insulin, you are not immune to this complication,* which is caused by too little insulin and too much sugar in your bloodstream.

Any diabetic can go into acidosis with continued poor control or a sudden stress such as an illness or injury. Not only that, but acidosis is not a benign complication. If it is allowed to progress into diabetic coma, it can endanger your health and even your life if it is untreated.

But acidosis has one virtue: it doesn't happen suddenly, except sometimes in a child, who has only a seventh of the fluid volume of an adult. It develops gradually, usually over a few days. Even in the case of some type 1 or brittle diabetics, it takes about 12 to 24 hours. High sugar and acetone will show up in your tests. This gives you time, if you are paying attention, to prevent serious consequences. If you make blood tests every day and have learned to recognize the symptoms, you will always know when you are in danger of acidosis and so you can take appropriate measures.

WHAT IS ACIDOSIS?

Acidosis or ketosis is a condition that results from hyper-glycemia, too *much* sugar in the blood because of too lit-tle insulin. In most cases, when the body lacks sufficient insulin to metabolize sugar, it starts burning its own fat tissue for fuel. The fat breakdown produces acetone and other ketones, fatty acids that are released into the bloodstream, changing its chemistry to an acid state.

If acidosis isn't checked, coma and eventually death are the end results. Acidosis is *serious*. Happily, the cur-rent emphasis on good control and frequent tests have made it a much less common event than it used to be.

THE WARNING SIGNS

You must act quickly as soon as you notice any signs of acidosis. What are the signs?

When your blood sugar increases without enough in-sulin to handle it, you will have the same symptoms that may have led you to the doctor when your diabetes was diagnosed. You will start spilling sugar into your urine. You will have to urinate frequently as the body tries to rid itself of the sugar, and you will soon become dehy-drated and extremely thirsty. Your skin will be dry. Your tongue will be dry. You may start to lose weight, your vi-sion may be dim or blurred. Your breath, because you are burning fat instead of carbohydrate, may smell fruity or sweet like peaches or violets or freshly mowed hay. You have trouble thinking straight.

Now, if you still don't acknowledge what's going on and deal with it, you will start to feel nauseated and per-haps develop abdominal pains. These symptoms will progress to a flushed face, labored breathing, drowsiness, disorientation, a rapid and weak pulse, low blood pressure, and eventually loss of consciousness.

WHAT CAUSES ACIDOSIS?

The most common causes of acidosis are omitting your insulin or oral hypoglycemic agent or having an infection. It can also be precipitated by poor control *whether or not you take insulin,* incorrect diet, failing to watch your blood-sugar levels with the proper vigilance and then not responding to high sugars immediately. *Preventing and dealing with abnormal sugar is a diabetic's Number One job.*

Sometimes you may not realize you are raising your blood sugar by eating too much of certain foods. In the summertime, for example, every doctor sees diabetics who have gone off the deep end with excessive amounts of fruit juices or raw fruits that are on their diet plan but not in the quantity in which they are consumed.

Illness, especially infection, dramatically increases your need for insulin, and is frequently the reason for an episode of high sugar and acidosis. *Be sure to take your insulin or pills when you are sick,* even though you are eating less or not at all. The fact is, you probably will need even *more* insulin, a situation you can judge only by making tests at regular close intervals. See Chapter 11 on coping with sick days.

Certain medications, such as prednisone, Dilantin, and protease inhibitors, can aggravate your diabetes, raising your blood sugar and causing you to require more insulin. These drugs can cause a condition usually seen only in elderly diabetics. It is called hyperosmolar nonketotic coma, with extremely high blood sugar but no acetone to tip you off in advance. Some of the newer psychotropic drugs for depression and anxiety have also been blamed for aggravating diabetes. So be sure your doctor takes your diabetes into account when prescribing any additional drugs. *This advice applies to all diabetics, whether or not you take insulin.*

Sometimes you may not be taking the right amount of insulin or oral agent; you can tell this from your test results and should report to your doctor. You may forget to take your medication, fail to get your proportions correct if you take split doses, use insulin whose potency has been affected by freezing or excessive heat.

But, no matter the reason for your high sugar and even if acidosis has already begun, you still have time to turn the tide.

By the way, don't take your pills with juice—it raises your blood sugar. Use water instead.

WHAT YOU SHOULD DO NOW

• Call your doctor the minute your tests show high sugar and acetone, or high sugar and the symptoms of thirst and urination.

• Check your blood *every two hours* when you see acetone.

• If your blood sugar and acetone tests are very high and you can't reach your doctor, take your usual dose of insulin plus an extra 5 or 10 units of Regular or fast-acting insulin such as Humalog, NovoLog, or Apidra every two hours. Don't wait. Do it now.

• Even if you don't normally take insulin, your doctor may prescribe 5 or 10 units of Regular or fast-acting insulin every two hours when your blood sugar is over 250 or so. That's a good reason to make sure you know how to give yourself a shot.

• Continue to make tests every two hours, and take additional Regular or other fast-acting insulin if your tests show high sugar and acetone.

• Do not *take extra insulin if your sugar is low even though your acetone is positive.* Now is the time to eat or drink carbohydrate to provide glucose for fuel.

• Rest, do not exercise.

• Drink as much water as you can to replace what you have lost.

• Keep in close touch with your doctor. Don't be afraid you're being a pest, because if you let yourself go into coma, you will be much more bother than you are now. Extreme acidosis requires that you go to the hospital for treatment.

• If your doctor recommends hospitalization, don't resist. Your sugar and acetone levels must be brought down to safety—fast.

REMEMBER THE THREE "T'S"

If you keep on top of your diabetes, you will never reach a state of serious acidosis or coma. In my many years of practice, with patients of all ages and all degrees of intelligence, I have rarely had to admit patients into the hospital for diabetic coma. That's because of the stress on tight control and three rigid rules:

1. Test your blood at least once a day; every two hours if you have high sugar and acetone.
2. Telephone your doctor.
3. Take extra insulin if you need it.

10

THE CHANCES OF DIABETIC COMPLICATIONS

If you live a good long life (and there's little reason today to expect you won't), you may eventually meet up with what is known as "diabetic complications." Diabetes is a metabolic condition with cumulative effects on the various systems of the body, so the longer you have it the more likely it is that you will have complications from it.

While that is true, there is strong evidence today that the incidence and severity of the complications are closely correlated with diabetic control. That's why you should know about these possible long-term effects right from the start, long before there is the slightest sign of them. It is vitally important, even crucial, to your future well-being to maintain your blood sugar at a normal or near-normal level as much of the time as you possibly can.

African Americans, especially women, not only have a higher incidence of diabetes but also are much more likely to suffer serious complications.

HIGH SUGAR TO BLAME

Consistently uncontrolled blood sugar causes diabetic complications. If you don't want to end up with long-term damage to almost every part of your body, you must be vigilant about your blood-glucose levels. Granted, that is not easy but it can be done.

The Diabetes Control and Complications Trial (DCCT) studied 1,441 type 1 diabetics in the United States and Canada from 1983 to 1993. The results showed that keeping blood-sugar levels close to normal slows the onset and progression of eye, kidney, and nerve diseases caused by diabetes. In fact, any sustained lowering of blood sugar helps prevent complications.

Among the volunteers, very tight sugar control plus attention to diet and exercise reduced the risk for developing retinopathy by 76 percent; prevented the development and slowed the progression of diabetic kidney disease by 50 percent; and lowered blood cholesterol by 35 percent, and diabetic neuropathy by 60 percent.

In another study, this time of 4,400 diabetics, those with blood-sugar levels consistently under 300 had three times less risk of complications after 15 years than those with higher levels. Those who kept their sugar below 255 had twenty times less risk. And for the volunteers with levels consistently below 120, the risk evaporated.

New research also links Alzheimer's disease and suggests that good control of blood sugar lowers the risk of developing this form of dementia.

THE OSTRICH SYNDROME

Unfortunately, many diabetic newcomers refuse to think about their unwelcome ailment and succumb to the "ostrich syndrome." As long as they don't have insulin reactions too often or land in the hospital with regularity, they think they're just fine. Meantime, they don't monitor their carbohydrate intake or check their blood, and the constant high level of sugar circulating throughout the tissues of their bodies is having its inexorable effect. This happens often with "mild" diabetics who, because they take little or no medication, think they needn't be concerned and test their blood very seldom.

While many diabetic complications can be adequately treated medically, it is obviously much better to avoid them in the first place if you can. The best way to do that is to remain as close as you can to ideal control, starting *early* in your life as a diabetic.

And, if you do begin to develop any of the typical complications, *get on their case promptly*. Picking them up early means avoiding many of the possible problems. If you wait until they have had a good start, reversing them may be difficult. Be sure your doctor watches for them and tests for them regularly. Don't be afraid to ask about complications or to insist on the proper checkups. Report any signs or symptoms the minute you notice them.

To some degree, diabetes eventually affects all the organs and systems of the body. Many of the medical problems of diabetics are no different from those that other people have, but occur more often and earlier. Some simply accelerate the natural aging process, especially in the large blood vessels and the connective tissue. But others are quite special to diabetes, and occur because of specific changes in the smaller blood vessels and nervous system. That's why it's important that your doctor is a diabetic specialist.

Much depends on the length of time you have had diabetes, the age you were when diagnosed, your race and your gender, and whether or not you must take insulin. Obviously, if you live long enough—diabetics tend to live to a ripe old age today—you are susceptible to more chronic problems, especially when you have a systemic condition. Besides, the longer you have diabetes, the more chance you have of acquiring any of the complications associated with it.

The more you know about diabetes, the fewer problems you will have, because you will understand the importance of tight control. Here are the pertinent facts about this collection of possible long-term diabetic complications.

YOU'RE PREDISPOSED TO HEART ATTACKS AND STROKES

Arteriosclerosis, narrowing of the large blood vessels, is to be expected by all of us as we grow older, and coronary heart disease is the single most common cause of death in the United States today. Diabetics certainly don't own exclusive rights to it, but they do comprise a disproportionate percentage of the population to have it. As a group, diabetics develop arteriosclerosis, especially in the heart, head, and legs, much more often and earlier—perhaps a decade or so—than nondiabetics.

It's been estimated by the United States Public Health Service that, while cardiovascular disease accounts for death among 50 percent of the general population, it is the cause of death for 75 percent of diabetics, who are twice as likely to have coronary heart disease, twice as likely to have strokes, and five times as likely to have arterial disease of the extremities. Women are particularly susceptible, and their chances of heart problems are about twice as high as for men.

One of the reasons for this situation is that diabetics have a predisposition toward hyperlipidemia, an abnormally high level of cholesterol circulating in the bloodstream rather than being stored. This leads to the accumulation of deposits of fatty substances on the inner walls of the major blood vessels. The thought today is that your genetic makeup, what you eat, and how efficient your insulin supply is, are all important factors.

People with diabetes tend to be overweight and to have high blood pressure, two conditions that can aggravate cardiovascular problems. Obesity requires an extra blood supply to nourish the extra body tissue, and puts its own strain on the heart as well. High blood pressure means an obvious stress on all the blood vessels, including the heart.

SO WHAT CAN YOU DO?

Since you know you have a tendency to develop cardiovascular complications earlier and more rapidly than other people, your job is to try to head them off. First, of course, as always, you must maintain excellent diabetic control, not just today and for a few days next month, but constantly. The less sugar circulating throughout your body the better.

If you are overweight, it is essential to lose weight. As you lose, you will see dramatic improvements in your blood cholesterol levels and—a most important feature— a drop in your blood pressure if it is high. Because high blood pressure always multiplies the risk of heart attack and stroke, you must bring it down with diet or, if necessary, medication.

Be sure your doctor is aware that you are diabetic. This may sound ridiculous—of course, your doctor knows—but if you use different doctors for different ailments, that may not be the case. Or they may forget for the moment.

WHY HYPERTENSION?

About 450 million years ago, there was a genetic change or mutation among some sea mammals that enabled a certain peptide to duplicate itself and form angiotensen, a substance that lines all of the blood vessels and increases blood pressure. This change enabled organisms to stand upright, rather than to swim or crawl on their bellies, and to live on land.

But it's too much of a good thing for human beings at the end of the evolutionary chain if too much angiotensen is produced, resulting in hypertension or high blood pressure. Fortunately, excessive angiotensen can now be countered with drugs like angiotensen-converting enzyme (ACE) inhibitors and angiotensin receptor blockers (ARBs).

DO YOURSELF A FAVOR

The biggest favor you can do yourself, if you want to live longer, is to get your blood pressure down to normal. The giraffe has the highest blood pressure of all the animals—about 240 mgs—and for a giraffe, that's fine, because the blood must be pumped all the way from its long legs up to its towering head. But *you* should be aiming for a blood pressure of 130/75 mm/Hg or lower. If you manage that, in addition to keeping your blood glucose under control and maintaining a healthy lipid profile, there's no telling how long you can live. Controlling your blood pressure also protects your kidneys and your eyes.

Most diabetics need drugs, usually more than one at a time, to make it happen. The preferred medications today include diuretics (water pills); angiotensin-converting enzyme inhibitors such as Altace or Capoten; angiotensin receptor blockers; beta blockers; and calcium channel blockers. By the way, the HOPE Study with Altace (ramipril) showed that in addition to lowering blood pressure, this drug decreased the incidence of diabetes, heart attacks, stroke, and kidney damage. Other drugs of the same class may well turn out to have the same effects, but they have not been studied enough yet to know for sure.

A BAD MATCH: DIABETES AND SMOKING

Smoking causes arterial spasms and raises blood pressure, so it is definitely a habit that must go. Diabetes and smoking combine to increase by many times the risk of heart disease. A diabetic, who already has a tendency toward coronary disease, needs to have everything going for him. Arterial spasms constrict the blood vessels, decreasing blood supply to the extremities—not a good idea, especially in your case. Besides, smoking may increase your chances of developing retinopathy and vision problems.

WATCH YOUR CHOLESTEROL

Because there is little controversy today over cholesterol's effect on your arteries, it is an excellent idea to limit the amount of saturated fats you eat and to increase the proportion of polyunsaturated varieties. If your cholesterol level is elevated, there are medications that your doctor may prescribe to help bring the lipid levels down to normal.

Your cholesterol level can be evaluated by the amount of high-density lipoproteins (HDL) it contains vs. the amount of low-density lipoproteins (LDL). The more high-density you have, the less chance there is that you will develop arteriosclerosis after age fifty. Exercise has been found to increase HDL, and so has an alcoholic drink or two before dinner. If your cholesterol value is below 150, it is not important to know what your HDL level is. It won't be high enough to matter. And if your cholesterol exceeds 350, it's too high to bother separating out. At this point, your HDL level is rarely sufficient to protect you from arteriosclerosis, and you are in dire need of reform.

DO-IT-YOURSELF CHOLESTEROL THERAPY

You can help improve your cholesterol profile by getting regular aerobic exercise, such as walking briskly for three miles, four times a week; losing weight if you are too heavy; quitting smoking; switching to monounsaturated fats and avoiding trans fats, formed when unsaturated oils are partly hydrogenated; drinking a moderate amount of alcohol every day; and sticking with the diet we have prescribed in this book. You might even try eating a lot of blueberries, reported by USDA researchers to contain a compound called pterostilbene that seems to break down cholesterol deposits.

But you should also start taking statins.

START THE STATINS

Ninety-five out of one hundred diabetes specialists, this one included, are convinced that *all* diabetics should take statins, even if their total cholesterol levels are not abnormally high and they're doing all the right things, for the simple reason that all diabetics have a higher risk of heart disease.

Statins have been around for about 20 years but have only recently become popular drugs. They were discovered in 1971 when a Japanese biochemist Akira Endo was searching for a new antibiotic. Knowing that many microorganisms require cholesterol for growth, he investigated HMG-COA reductase inhibitor derived from a penicillium mold and discovered that it lowered cholesterol. Later, other statins were developed from other molds, but the newest varieties are synthetic derivatives.

LOWER YOUR LDL

The statin drugs on the market today are designed to reduce the level of LDL, the "bad" cholesterol that clogs arteries. Current data indicate that they are safe except for children under ten, women who are pregnant or nursing, and others who have liver problems or are taking other drugs that can combine with statins to cause liver damage. Your liver function should be tested before you start the daily regime and periodically thereafter, because, though rare, a person may develop liver damage. And if you have unexplained muscle pain or weakness, especially combined with a fever, report it to your doctor immediately because it could indicate a serious problem.

The goal is to get your LDL below 100 mg/dl, or preferably 70, if you are a diabetic with hypertension or heart disease.

The LDL-lowering drugs include lovastatin (generic, Mevacor), atorvastatin (Lipitor), fluvastatin (Lescol), pravastatin (Pravachol), rosuvastatin (Crestor), and simvastatin (Zocor). Lipitor and Crestor are the most potent, with Crestor the best at raising HDL. But take care: high doses of over 40 mgs a day could give you liver problems.

If you are taking the highest effective dose and you need even more help getting your LDL to an acceptable level, a different kind of cholesterol-cutting drug—ezetimibe (Zetia)—can be added to it. Zetia helps block the absorp-

tion of cholesterol from food. There is even a combination drug, Vytorin, that combines Zocor and Zetia in one
pill. In 2005, the FDA gave the green light for Lipitor to
be prescribed to lower the stroke risk rate in type 2 diabetics even if they do not yet show evidence of heart disease.

If a particular statin isn't right for you or if it doesn't
do the job, the first choice is to change to another that
does not go through the usual pathway. Or you can
switch to one of the bile-acid-binding resins, such as
cholestyramine (Pravalite and Questran Light), cole-
sevelam (Welchol), or colestipol (Colestid).

RAISE YOUR HDL

While LDL levels should be low, the opposite is true of
HDL. The higher your HDL the better. Men should have
a level of at least 40 mg/dl, while women must try for a
minimum of 50 mg/dl. HDL, known as the "good" cholesterol, acts as an arterial Roto-Rooter that clears cholesterol out of the arteries, acts as an anti-inflammatory
agent and antioxidant, and has important anticlotting
properties.

Statins don't do much for HDL, but other drugs do.
The most effective are the niacin-based medications
such as Niaspan and a new drug, still under development, called Torcetrapid that can dramatically raise
HDL when combined with Lipitor.

REDUCE THOSE TRIGLYCERIDES

A third variety of blood fats is triglyceride and, like
LDL, it should be at the lowest possible level, no higher
than 150 mg/dl or close to it.

For many years, Lopid was the only drug available to deal with high triglyceride levels and was often given together with statins. But a few other medications, all fibrates, have come along. One newcomer is Antara, a fibrate used in Europe for many years, which reduces triglycerides along with LDL, and even raises HDL slightly. Another is TriCor, which has good results on both LDL and triglycerides. The latest drug developed for this purpose is Omacor, a concentrated form of the omega-3 oils found in some fatty fish. It has been shown to produce significant drops in people with triglyceride levels as high as 500 mg/dl.

By the way, Lopid taken alone is fine, but do not take it in combination with the oral agents Avandia or Actos, both TZDs, because Lopid may increase their strength. In addition, don't take it with TriCor because it increases your chances of muscle aches.

BEWARE OF GRAPEFRUIT

Don't take a statin drug within an hour or two of eating grapefruit or drinking grapefruit juice because they can block liver enzymes that break down and clear drugs from the body. When you take a statin or a few other medications, such as calcium channel blockers and some antihistamines and tranquilizers, eating grapefruit is like taking a higher dose, because grapefruit intensifies the drug's effects.

ARE REACTIONS HARMFUL?

If you already have arteriosclerosis, you should do your best to avoid insulin reactions. That's because severe reactions are thought to put additional stress on the already narrowed blood vessels supplying the heart or the brain. However, this isn't as important as doctors have thought in the past. In fear of shocks, they have often allowed their patients to consistently spill too much sugar. Today the thinking is that reactions do not pose a great danger and that it is much more important to control blood sugar closely, even with the risk of a few reactions. In the long run, tight control is best.

GET YOUR EXERCISE

Next, exercise. Everyone's cardiovascular system benefits from regular exercise, especially exercise that gets the heart pumping and the lungs expanding. If you get enough (always under the supervision of your doctor), you can significantly lower your risk of heart attack. Exercise can slow your heart rate, lower your blood pressure, help burn up calories, cut down LDL levels, raise HDL, and as an added bonus, help keep your diabetes under control by allowing you to handle carbohydrates more efficiently.

THE ASPIRIN TREATMENT

Most diabetologists recommend a daily dose of aspirin to help ward off heart problems because of its anticlotting effect.

It won't hurt to take one low-dose aspirin (81 mgs) a day. Check with your physician first, however. If you have retinopathy associated with hemorrhaging, or a tendency toward bleeding ulcers, it is *not* a good idea to take even a low-dose aspirin regularly.

THE CHANCES OF EYE PROBLEMS

There was a time, not long ago, when all diabetics had a good chance of developing serious vision problems, but that has drastically changed in recent years. Though it is true that diabetes is still the leading cause of blindness, there is an excellent chance it's not going to happen to you. And the odds are improving in your favor every day because of new research and treatments.

Today we have sophisticated methods of coping with the typical diabetic eye changes. And we know that, with good diabetic control, especially in the first five years, you are much less likely to develop eventual difficulties. There are exceptions to every rule, of course, but, in general, people whose blood sugars are kept consistently below a certain level tend to show many fewer complications of all kinds.

Type 2 diabetics are not as likely to develop serious eye changes as those who have type 1 that usually strikes in childhood; African Americans are in a higher risk category; and people treated by diet alone or oral agents have less chance of eye complications than those who are dependent on insulin.

Nine out of ten diabetics eventually show some vascular changes in their retinas, the linings of the backs of the eyes where light is received and then sent to the brain for interpretation. Called background or nonproliferative retinopathy, these early changes usually appear and then stay pretty much as they are. Of the 90 percent of those diabetics who develop background retinopathy, just one in five will progress to the next set of complications called proliferative retinopathy or retinitis proliferans. This is a more precarious situation, but even among people in this group, blindness can, in most cases, be prevented.

So, while this is definitely a concern, it is not inevitable and it gives you an excellent reason to keep your blood-sugar levels within acceptable boundaries. Temporary lapses into high levels, which happen to everyone, aren't what we are talking about. It is the consistent lack of tight control that is much more likely to cause trouble later in your life.

You, as a diabetic, are also at risk for other eye diseases. For example, you are nearly twice as likely to get glaucoma as other adults, and this risk increases the longer you've had diabetes. Cataracts, too, are twice as prevalent among diabetics and tend to develop at an earlier age.

BACKGROUND RETINOPATHY

The retina is nourished by a network of tiny capillaries. After many years of diabetes, the walls or the basement membranes of these minuscule blood vessels become damaged because of high blood sugar and high blood pressure, cutting down the oxygen supply to the eyes. They may then become weakened and form little bulges called microaneurysms. These, like any balloons, tend to have fragile walls and may leak serum inside the retina, sometimes causing macular edema—swelling from the leaking fluid. Sometimes, too, the tiny capillaries rupture and little hemorrhages occur in the backs of the eyes.

The doctor who examines your eyes looks for these microaneurysms, which show up as red dots, as well as small collections of soft, cottony or yellowish fatty materials, which are actually cholesterol deposits and are called exudates. If you have them, you have background retinopathy, which does not mean things will get worse.

This will probably become merely a chronic condition, which your diabetologist and ophthalmologist must check periodically. You probably will not even be aware of it and it will not affect your vision unless it occurs around the macula, a very small area responsible for your central vision.

WHAT'S TO BE DONE ABOUT IT?

The very first thing you can do about retinopathy and your diabetes is to stop denying the truth. If you don't maintain very good control over your blood-sugar levels, you are issuing an invitation to a great many problems. Numerous studies have conclusively shown that sugar levels are closely linked with eye changes, all of them pointing to the importance of keeping the sugar within the normal range (below 100 mgs fasting and below 140 mgs two hours after eating), therefore keeping your HbA1c below 6 percent.

This is not to say that maintaining perfect control (which is impossible anyway) over many years will absolutely ward off eye complications. Some people take excellent care of themselves and keep their blood sugars very close to normal, yet still develop retinopathy, while others who are wildly out of control never have it. But, as a rule, the majority of diabetics who maintain good control will not have retinopathy, while the majority of those who do not monitor their sugar levels carefully will develop eye complications. This includes *all* diabetics on insulin, oral agents, or even diet alone.

The second thing you can do if you have background retinopathy is to be sure your blood pressure is within the normal range. Hypertension, even without diabetes, can cause retinopathy because the little blood vessels in the eyes are under stress. The combination of the two ailments obviously is highly undesirable. And, since smokers have a higher incidence of retinopathy, smoking, for this among many other reasons, is not acceptable for you as a diabetic.

AN EYE CHECKUP EVERY THREE MONTHS

Be certain your physician examines your eyes at *every* visit (diabetics should see their doctors at least every three months), and *remind* the doctor, if necessary, to do so. If this chore doesn't seem very important to the person you have chosen as your physician, it might be a good idea to find another. The minute the doctor sees signs of retinopathy, you should promptly see an ophthalmologist (an M.D. with a specialty in ophthalmology—not an optician or an optometrist) and then return for checkups *at least* every six months.

In fact, you should see this specialist initially just after your diagnosis as a diabetic, especially if you have the type 2 variety of diabetes. You may have had asymptomatic diabetes for years before the diagnosis and it is an excellent idea to check out your eyes now.

Even without any eye changes, it's most important to see the ophthalmologist at least once a year. Do not wait for any sudden decreased vision or strange symptoms to make your first appointment, or even for your doctor to see evidence of microaneurysms. With the use of a special fluorescent dye, diabetic eye changes can be discovered by a specialist even earlier.

There are no obvious symptoms in the early stages of retinopathy, and it is not at all uncommon to have excellent vision at the time the condition is diagnosed, even though the damage has already begun. By the time you notice any visual problems, it may be too late to remedy the situation. So don't procrastinate—make that appointment now.

In addition to those regular visits to your ophthalmologist, it is an excellent idea to schedule an appointment with a retinal specialist at least every year after your fifth year as a diabetic. General doctors, or even diabetologists, cannot be relied upon to detect early changes. It's important to catch eye problems such as retinopathy and glaucoma as early as possible before your vision is impaired.

Meanwhile, lower your cholesterol level if it is out of the normal range.

PROLIFERATIVE RETINOPATHY EXPLAINED

Retinitis proliferans is more serious than background retinopathy and it's important to know that if treatment is going to be useful, you must start *early.* That means *right now,* just as soon as it is diagnosed. A study of 847 cases of retinitis proliferans at the Joslin Clinic, in which I was a principal investigator, showed that it takes 17.4 years, on average, for a youngster with type 1 diabetes who is going to have this condition to develop it; and 4.3 years, on the average, for a person over sixty. Your doctor should be aware of the natural history of this complication.

Only about 40 percent of people who already have retinitis proliferans report to their physicians that they have noticed changes in vision or are experiencing symptoms like streaks or flashes. This means the other 60 percent with serious eye changes are not getting the signals or are not acknowledging them. That is why it is vital for your doctor always to check the backs of your eyes.

Retinitis proliferans is a serious situation. It works like this: the capillaries along the inner surfaces of the retina start multiplying or proliferating, probably as a response to decreased oxygen supply to the eye. These new blood vessels try to bring more oxygen into the area, just as fire hoses bring water to a fire, but they are very fragile. They break easily and then may bleed into the retina and the vitreous, the gel-like substance that fills the eyeball. This makes the vitreous murky, preventing the passage of light from the lens to the retina. Fortunately, the blood is often reabsorbed spontaneously and the vitreous clears again.

In some cases of retinitis proliferans, the rapid growth of new and delicate blood vessels and the resulting bleeding stimulates the formation of fibrous scar tissue that may contract and cause a detached retina. Retinitis proliferans can also lead to a form of glaucoma that can be difficult to treat.

All of this usually comes about quite slowly. If the proliferation happens only on the periphery of the retina and the vitreous isn't clouded, vision won't be seriously affected. But if it covers the central portion of the retina, if the retina starts to detach, or if the vitreous becomes opaque, then we have problems. But even then, we have some solutions.

LASER BEAMS AND MORE

Several good treatments have been developed and perfected in recent years, with others on the way. One of these is photocoagulation, which involves the use of a laser aimed at the leaking or abnormally proliferating blood vessels. The beam, which is usually painless, destroys the unwanted fragile capillaries and seals them off, resulting in harmless scar tissue. The laser is also used to shoot pinpoint blasts around the periphery of leaky eye tissue, closing off these outer capillaries to decrease the eye's oxygen requirements. Now more of the available blood will go to the central and most important area of the retina. Sometimes, the laser beam is used to glue the retina back in place if it is detached or in danger of becoming detached. Photocoagulation has become a major tool of the ophthalmologist and often manages to stop retinal damage right in its tracks. Lasers can also treat diabetic glaucoma.

A procedure called *vitrectomy* is another important new treatment for eyes seriously affected by retinitis proliferans. If the vitreous inside the eyeball has become clouded with little bits of leaking blood, or if it has started to contract because of the bleeding and to pull on the retina, threatening to detach it, this technique may be employed to improve the situation. A special precision instrument is used to bore a tiny hole into the eye and suction out the stained vitreous, at the same time replacing it with clear saline solution. This procedure can not only eliminate the clouded vision, but it can also give the ophthalmologist an opportunity to see into your eyes and evaluate the usefulness of laser treatment.

NEWCOMERS ON THE BLOCK

Although laser treatments and vitrectomies have been godsends for diabetics with retinopathy, even better ways of remedying the damage have come along. Cortisone injections, for example, can reduce inflammation and are frequently used today.

Even more promising are the drugs that inhibit the action of VEGF (vegetative endothelial growth factor), a substance that encourages the formation of fragile new blood vessels in the retina. The first VEGF blockers to be developed must be injected directly into the eyes, something nobody cares to contemplate, but taken orally, it is feared that they could compromise the blood supply to the heart and feet, which is something diabetics don't need.

Macugen, on the market since 2005, was the first approved drug for this purpose and is also used to treat macular degeneration. It is injected once every four weeks. Clinical trials show that a second variety, Lucentis, now awaiting approval, may turn out to be even more effective. An altered version of Avastin, a cancer drug that chokes off the blood supply to tumors, Lucentis is also injected once a month. And Arxxant (roboxitaurin) inhibits VEGF and has shown some benefit for macular edema but has not yet been as successful as hoped in preventing the formation of new blood vessels. Meanwhile, a pill called Squalamine, derived from shark liver oil and designed to affect only the blood vessels in the eyes and nowhere else, is in the works at Johns Hopkins Medical School.

WILL VITAMIN C HELP?

Though vitamin C in combination with rutin was once widely prescribed for retinopathy, studies have shown that rutin isn't absorbed by the body at all, and the effectiveness of vitamin C as a way to strengthen the capillary walls is still being debated. In other words, nobody knows for sure whether it will help prevent retinopathy, or colds either for that matter. Our theory is, though, that it can't hurt to take about 500 mgs of C every day. The best that could happen is that it works; the worst is that it doesn't. Excess vitamin C is excreted in the urine.

WHAT ABOUT MAGNESIUM?

A study comparing three groups of diabetics found the lowest amount of magnesium in those with the greatest degree of retinopathy. And recent research suggests that people with the highest levels of magnesium in their diets have the lowest risk of getting diabetes. Since magnesium can be found in such foods as whole grains, cereals, beans, and nuts, you probably don't need a supplement. On the other hand, the magnesium level of your blood is easily tested, and if it turns out to be low, a supplement couldn't hurt.

MY VISION IS BLURRY. IS THAT BAD?

Not necessarily. Your vision can be affected simply by your current blood-sugar level. If the level is high or fluctuating, your sight may be fuzzy, out of focus. It will clear up when you're once more under good control, though it may take anywhere from a few days to a few weeks. *Nevertheless, always go to your diabetic specialist when your vision changes in any way.*

Blurred vision is *expected* when your diabetes is first diagnosed and you are treated with insulin for the first time. After undergoing a week or two of insulin therapy and having your blood sugar go down to an acceptable level, you may find you cannot focus clearly. Don't panic. It will get better before long.

Probably the blurred vision occurs because, during the period of poor control and dehydration, the eyes gradually lost some of their fluid content as well as fluids from the rest of the body, altering their shape. In addition, the increased sugar content in the eyes' lenses may cause them to swell and alter their refraction of light. As both these factors swing back toward normal, you will notice the blurriness until you adjust once more.

By the way, be sure your sugar is in optimum control *before* you go to the ophthalmologist for new eyeglasses. If your sugar is high, your distance vision may be affected. If it is very low, your near vision may change. So new glasses that are fitted today may not be right for you tomorrow or next week. If you are a new diabetic, wait at least a month after you have been stabilized before going for a new prescription.

WHAT CAUSES DOUBLE VISION?

Very low blood-sugar levels can temporarily produce double vision. If the two images persist, however, it may be due to infarction of a nerve of the eye muscles and an uneven pull of the muscles. If an eye is pulled off-center unilaterally, you will see two images, a decidedly unpleasant phenomenon. But don't worry, it usually disappears spontaneously within three to six weeks in just about every case, and all you'll need is an eye patch until it does.

DO DIABETICS HAVE MORE CATARACTS?

They do. They also tend to get them at an earlier age and the progression is more rapid. Cataracts include both the "snowflake" metabolic variety that occasionally occurs in type 1 diabetics and the "senile" kind that is part of the normal aging process.

Treatment for cataracts is the same for everyone, though for diabetics the doctors may decide on surgery at a slightly earlier stage of development in order to have an opportunity to examine the back of the retina.

With cataract surgery, as with any other kind of operation, it is very important to be under optimum control when you have the procedure so that healing will be normal and infections more easily avoided.

A lens implant at the time of surgery will not interfere with laser treatment if you ever require it at a later time.

DO DIABETICS HAVE MORE GLAUCOMA?

Yes, and the longer they have had diabetes, the greater the risk of developing it. It's important to catch glaucoma early so it can be treated with medications and/or laser or other forms of surgery before it impairs your vision. Glaucoma develops slowly and insidiously without any obvious symptoms. Half of those who have it don't even know it.

ARE CONTACT LENSES SAFE?

There is no reason you cannot wear contact lenses if the outer surfaces of your eyes are in healthy condition. Be sure, however, to go to a reputable ophthalmologist who has extensive experience in fitting contacts.

SHOULD I WORRY ABOUT "FLOATERS"?

Floaters or "flying mice," as they have been dubbed, are little pieces of protein that you can see fleetingly as they float through the vitreous, the gel-like fluid within the eyeball. These are nothing to be concerned about unless they develop suddenly or are accompanied by flashes of light (in which case, see your ophthalmologist immediately to make sure the retina is not torn). Most people have floaters, though diabetics seem to have them more often than others.

THE EFFECTS OF MARIJUANA

Marijuana lowers the pressure within the eyeball, so it is theoretically possible that it may encourage bleeding of the fragile capillaries of the retina. This is a good reason, along with a few others, not to use it. It encourages a desire for sweets among some people, which diabetics can't afford, and tends to alter the sense of time. You may forget to eat on time and then have a serious insulin reaction.

THE EFFECTS OF EXERCISE

Regular vigorous exercise helps to prevent retinopathy and other diabetic complications although you should never lift weights above your eye level if you are diabetic. But the story is quite different if you already have retinopathy. Now it's important *not* to raise your blood pressure, which can trigger more hemorrhaging of those tiny blood vessels in the backs of the eyes. Don't do anything strenuous without consulting your doctor, and don't even think of lifting weights.

DIABETES AND YOUR EARS

Consider getting a yearly hearing test because if you have diabetes, and especially if you have hypertension, you're more likely to suffer earlier and faster hearing loss. This is probably because of impeded blood flow to the auditory nerves.

COPING WITH KIDNEY PROBLEMS

Because your two kidneys—which are each about the size of your fist and located near the middle of your back just below the rib cage, are intricate filters with the important job of eliminating waste products and excess water from the blood while holding on to certain vital proteins—it is very important that they continue to function smoothly. Kidney complications, however, can be one of the problems that beset long-time diabetics, especially African American diabetics, among whom chronic kidney problems due to this disease are almost three times greater than among whites.

Diabetes is America's leading cause of kidney failure because of a tendency for all of the blood vessels in the body to weaken and for the walls or basement membranes of the kidneys' complex network of capillaries to thicken and, at the same time, become too porous. These incredibly complicated filters then allow a loss of proteins—albumin and globulin—into the urine. Further progression can result in uremia and kidney failure, which can be treated only by dialysis or kidney transplants.

Other factors that can lead to kidney complications are high blood pressure and urinary infections, problems diabetics are prone to have. That's why early and vigorous treatment of infections is very important and why blood-pressure control is vital. Half of all diabetics have hypertension, and this combination leads to both heart and kidney disease. In fact, 40 to 50 percent of type 2s with early kidney damage, called microalbuminaria, eventually die of cardiovascular disease.

DETECTING EARLY KIDNEY PROBLEMS

If you've lived many years with high blood-sugar levels, especially when combined with high blood pressure, you may eventually develop microalbuminurea—tiny amounts of the protein albumin leak into the urine—an early warning sign that you are at risk of more serious difficulties. Standard urine tests can detect a level of 300 mgs of albumin, but they are not sensitive enough to detect amounts smaller than that. The first red flag goes up at much lower levels, however, perhaps even at 30 mgs, so make sure your doctor ordes a microalbumin test and a check of urinary creatinine levels *at least once a year.*

The ADA recommends starting to screen for microalbuminuria in those who have had type 1 diabetes for five years, and at the time of diagnosis in people with type 2. But testing for microalbuminuria alone may miss many cases of kidney disease, so especially for type 2s, experts now recommend also testing the glomerular filtration rate (GFR) and creatinine clearance, which are indications of how well the kidneys are able to filter waste from the blood. A buildup of creatinine and blood urea nitrogen (BUN) in the bloodstream is a sign that kidney function is beginning to decline.

Another important weapon is the HbA1c test (see page 173). It measures glucose levels over a two- or three-month period and can be an indication of your risk for diabetic complications.

TREATING KIDNEY PROBLEMS

In addition to tight control of your glucose, the initial treatment if you are spilling albumin in your urine is usually a diuretic such as diazide, along with lifestyle changes—losing weight, cutting down on salt and alcohol, getting more exercise, and perhaps even including soy protein supplements.

But you will probably do better with a combination of two drugs that are commonly used to lower blood pressure but that also tend to protect the kidneys: ACE (angiotensin-converting enzyme) inhibitors such as Altace or Capoten, and ARBs (angiotensin receptor blockers). These medications are so effective that virtually everyone with diabetes should probably start taking them even before kidney disease develops. In most cases, taking both of these drugs will raise the chances of preserving kidney function. ACE inhibitors, however, sometimes cause a cough. If that happens to you, you should immediately switch to an ARB alone.

More sophisticated treatments include calcium channel blockers in addition to the ACE inhibitors, and beta blockers to control hypertension and its deleterious effects on the kidneys.

There's promise, too, of another mode of defense against kidney failure with the use of new compounds such as aminoguanadine, glycosaminoglycans, and Arxxant (roboxistaurin). Used early on, they seem to help prevent "advance glycation end products," which is the attachment of glucose to the kidneys, causing them to become waterlogged and thickened.

BEWARE OF ANALGESICS

If analgesics—aspirin, acetaminophen, ibuprofen, ketoprofen, and naproxen—are taken in excess or over a long period of time, they can harm your kidneys. If you have diabetes, and especially if you already show signs of renal damage, it's best not to use them without checking with your physician.

THE WEIRD EFFECTS OF NEUROPATHY

Neuropathy, probably the most common as well as the strangest of all the possible diabetic complications, affects nerve function and isn't very well understood even today. Its symptoms can be mild and simply an annoyance, or they can make life pretty miserable. The only good thing about neuropathy is that its weird effects sometimes disappear or improve dramatically after a while. This can take from a couple of months to a couple of years. Although diabetes is the most common cause of neuropathy, it can also be the result of autoimmune diseases, compression problems, certain vitamin deficiencies, drugs, alcoholism, and toxic substances. Or it can be a complete mystery, its cause unknown.

Because neuropathy is nerve damage that interferes with the ability of the nerves to conduct messages and at times actually alters them, sometimes it results in outright severe pain, sometimes in tingling, a pins-and-needles sensation, burning, itching, weakness, or simply numbness. Occasionally there will be pain and numbness at the same time. These symptoms, which can show up in many parts of the body, come and go unpredictably, though for most people they tend to be decidedly worse at night. And they often confound the doctors, who may diagnose them as something else.

Nobody knows just why neuropathy happens, but research indicates that the "sorbitol pathway" may be at the bottom of it. When sugar persistently circulates at high levels in the body tissues, certain enzymes turn the glucose into fructose, then into sorbitol. Sorbitol, a sugar that cannot return to its previous incarnations as glucose and fructose, causes damage to the nerve endings so they are unable to carry on their normal metabolism and consequently their normal function. Sorbitol taken by mouth, however, does not affect the nerves.

PERIPHERAL NEUROPATHY

Neuropathy most often affects the legs and feet, and sometimes the hands, where it gives you pain or tingling, or the odd impression of walking on sand or pebbles. This is called peripheral neuropathy. Often there's a *lack* of sensation, so it feels as if you are walking on wood or even on pillows or clouds. Some people say it feels as if their feet do not belong to them. Others have pain and lack of sensation at the very same time, and some become extraordinarily sensitive to touch so that even the weight of sheets is a torment. The pain may be constant or intermittent, usually becoming much more troublesome at night. Often it occurs *only* at night, disappearing when the sun comes up. Cold, wet weather seems to aggravate it.

If you haven't much feeling in your feet, you will now have to be especially careful not to injure them without realizing it, and to keep an eye out for infections you can't feel. See Chapter 12 for a complete discussion of foot care.

If you have neuropathic pain, take comfort in the fact that it may get better in a few months. In fact, some specialists say the worse the pain, the faster it goes away, leaving some numbness in its place. Meantime, you may need painkillers or tranquilizers to help you sleep.

TREATING PERIPHERAL NEUROPATHY

Because not much is known about what actually causes neuropathy, not much is known about what to do about it either. In some cases, medication can be helpful. In others, the symptoms disappear as mysteriously as they came, and most usually go away eventually or markedly improve.

In the early stages, 100 mgs of vitamin B_1 taken daily can be effective. If it isn't, try B_{12} injections up to 20 units. If you wish, you can inject this along with your insulin.

Work is now under way to test the effectiveness of a drug called myonisotol in increasing nerve conduction. This is a substance found in the nerve coverings, and also in cantaloupes and peanuts. On the chance this natural form may help you, test it out by eating a quarter of a cantaloupe in place of other vitamin C fruits in the morning.

If your neuropathy is troublesome, you and your doctor will have to come up with medication that works for you. Unfortunately, no medication eases the discomfort for everyone so you may have to keep trying one after the other. Sharp pains may respond to carbamazepine (Tegretol). Some people are helped by applying capsaicin (Zostrex) to the skin two to four times a day. If you use capsaicin, keep your hands away from your eyes after you use it—it is made of red pepper and it stings. Or try Lidocain, also applied to the skin, either as a cream or a patch.

A drug called Tolrestat, used in other countries but not yet in the United States, seems to improve autonomic function, and electrical spinal cord stimulation (ESCS) has been found in tests to help some people whose symptoms do not respond to other treatments.

There is also some evidence that evening primrose oil, otherwise known as alpha lipoic acid and sold in health-food stores, may provide relief in doses of 500 mgs three times a day.

TAKING THE EDGE OFF THE PAIN

The big news in the treatment of neuropathy is a group of medications that, although they won't cure or even improve the condition, can dull the discomfort caused by the damaged nerve endings. Neurontin (gabapentin), an anticonvulsant, is probably the one most commonly prescribed and has long been considered the drug of choice for neuropathy. But a couple of others are now competing for that role.

Cymbalta (duloxetine), an antidepressant, the first drug specifically approved by the FDA for this use, alleviates the discomfort for many people with neuropathy. Its side effects include nausea, increased sweating, and dizziness.

Lyrica (pregabalin), even newer, is similar to Neurontin but acts more quickly and perhaps more effectively. Like everything else, it too has possible side effects, such as dizziness, sleepiness, and weight gain.

A drug called Lumeron has demonstrated some encouraging results but is still undergoing clinical trials, as is Epalrestat, an aldose reductase inhibitor, which is reported to show promising results in delaying the progression of diabetic neuropathy as well as retina and kidney damage.

CAUTION: Never quit taking any of these drugs abruptly because sudden withdrawal can cause some disturbing and perhaps even dangerous problems. Tapering off is the way to go.

THE SORBITOL CONNECTION

A new theory about neuropathy is that it is caused by an enzyme called aldose reductase that turns excessive amounts of glucose circulating in the bloodstream into sorbitol, a type of sugar alcohol, resulting in stress and damage to the nerves. Aldose reductase inhibitors, such as the medications Fiderestat and Ranirestat, are being studied as potential treatments for nerve damage, perhaps even reversing the progression of neuropathy.

Meanwhile, exercise regularly, don't smoke, limit alcohol to only a few drinks a week, and inspect your feet and legs daily. And let's not forget *control*. Obviously, good control over your blood-sugar level may help you avoid the neuropathies in the first place. And it is quite possible it can prevent further progress of problems you already have.

NOTE: if you have been in poor control for a long time, have developed neuropathy, but now seek tight control, you may find that any neuropathic discomforts are aggravated at first. This may tempt you to revert to your old bad habits. But hold on. If you stay with it, you will soon feel better.

NEUROPATHIC FOOT ULCERS

Because neuropathy often causes a lack of feeling on the bottoms of the feet, it's possible to develop sores, usually at pressure points, that you are unaware of. This causes calluses that then put more pressure on the area. Eventually, unnoticed, a neuropathic ulcer may form beneath the calluses, becoming infected and leading to serious trouble if it is unchecked.

See Chapter 12 for advice on avoiding this kind of

foot problem before it starts. Once an ulcer develops, it must be treated immediately and vigorously if you don't want to be in for a long siege. The infection must be drained and a course of antibiotics begun *promptly*. Then the pressure must be relieved by staying off your feet or by using special pads in your shoes.

Because of the potential seriousness of an ulcer, your feet must be examined constantly by you and periodically by both your doctor and your podiatrist.

OTHER NEUROPATHIC HAUNTS

Though the feet are neuropathy's favorite targets, it can affect other parts of you, too. Occasionally people find their hands become somewhat insensitive, almost as if they are wearing gloves. Sometimes the muscles of the hands diminish in size, or the muscles between the fingers become atrophied, making it difficult to use the hands for small movements such as buttoning a shirt. The same sort of phenomenon sometimes occurs in the feet when the muscles at the base of the toes weaken, resulting in pressure and ulcers on the metatarsal pads.

Diabetics also sometimes develop a condition called Dupuytren's contracture. The tendons of the palm of the hand become thickened and shortened, hindering mobility. Surgery can correct these "frozen" hands.

Occasionally neuropathy affects the muscles of the eyes, causing double vision and perhaps sharp pain. The prognosis is usually excellent for double vision, with complete recovery within about six weeks.

The gastrointestinal tract is another part of the body that may be affected by this strange nerve damage peculiar to diabetes. The esophagus and stomach, as well as the intestines, may not contract with their usual vigor, with the result that they don't empty efficiently. The delay may affect your diabetic control by slowing down the absorption of food. Or it may cause bloating, heartburn, reflux, erratic glucose levels, or perhaps nausea or lack of appetite. It often helps this gastroparesis to cut back on the fat and fiber in your diet, eat five or six small meals a day, or go on a liquid diet temporarily, and to take Reglan, a drug that speeds up intestinal peristalsis.

Some people with intestinal neuropathy find they develop diarrhea at unpredictable moments, most often at night. Or they become severely constipated. About half of those with diabetic diarrhea respond well to antibiotics, such as erythromycin, that work on the intestinal bacteria. Other people get good results from antidiarrhea medications such as Lomotil or codeine. The constipation usually responds to laxatives or stool softeners. Keep in mind that fatigue and stress have a poor effect on bowel problems.

Most important of all, try to maintain very good blood-glucose control, which may involve frequent glucose monitoring and additional insulin injections.

URINARY PROBLEMS

The bladder may also be affected by this strange villain if the nerve damage interferes with its ability to contract, or with its owner's ability to sense when it is full and needs emptying. The urine may back up into the kidneys or the bladder may not empty completely, providing a happy home for bacteria and infections. Sometimes drugs such as Hytrin, Cardura, Detrol, or Uroxatral can improve this organ's muscle tone and its ability to empty.

Because constant urinary infections that may hang on

stubbornly can eventually lead to serious kidney dis-function, all diabetics must be sure to watch closely for them. If you have any symptoms of an infection, such as burning, pain, or urgency, see your doctor immediately. Make certain you are given the proper tests to determine the right drugs to combat it, and that you stay on the drugs until the infection is totally destroyed. If you have a tendency to get infections, your doctor should check for them by examining your urine under a microscope at every examination (at least every three months), *whether or not* you have symptoms.

If you're a woman, make sure to drink a lot of water before and after sex to keep the infection rate down. And always wipe yourself from front to back.

If you notice you are not urinating very often and, when you do, you produce a less-than-expected amount, discuss this with your doctor, who may suggest that you urinate every few hours on schedule rather than wait for the urge, or may prescribe drugs to stimulate urination. On the other hand, if you tend to urinate often but little is coming out, it may indicate paresis of the bladder that is causing retention. Again, don't keep this information to yourself. Bring it up at your next visit.

THE RARER NEUROPATHIES

A few other neuropathic effects include:

• Orthostatic hypotension, which is temporary low pressure occurring when you stand or sit up suddenly or raise your head. This makes you lightheaded, dizzy, and sometimes unsteady on your feet for a few moments. Medication such as Midodrine can help, along with support hose to help constrict the blood vessels in the legs.

• Abnormal sweating may be a form of neuropathy,

especially when it appears on the face (or *half* the face) after eating.

• "Dry foot," when the feet don't produce sweat and so tend to dry out and crack. Or the opposite, feet that are particularly sweaty.

• Radicular pain, a sharp abdominal pain that usually recedes after a while.

• Charcot's foot, a phenomenon that is frequently triggered by neuropathy. It usually starts with painless fractures of the bones of the foot and progresses if untreated to muscle atrophy and joint damage until the foot loses its normal anatomy and becomes deformed. Treatment is to catch the problem early, stay off your feet, and wear special footwear.

• Sexual impotence after many years of diabetes, and retrograde ejaculation, which means the semen flows back into the bladder rather than out of the penis (see Chapter 14).

DIABETES AND YOUR TEETH

No doubt you'd like to keep a complete set of your very own teeth forever—nobody looks forward to dropping his teeth into a glass every night. If so, you are going to have to take extraordinarily good care of them, because you are three or four times more susceptible than most people to gum and bone disease, the major cause of tooth loss. That is another result of the effect of high blood sugar on the body's myriad tiny capillaries. The thickened walls of the little blood vessels make oxygen-vs.-waste exchange less efficient. And you are then more likely to develop infections that are difficult to get rid of.

If your diabetes is poorly controlled, your white blood cells, whose job it is to fight off bacteria, are less effective in their battle against infection, causing it to become more severe and harder to heal. The reason is that the white cells don't migrate as quickly as they should to the source of the infection and, once there, are not as vigorous in their battle against the offending bacteria. Because there is a close correlation between blood sugar and periodontal disease, the best way to prevent problems is to maintain tight control of your sugar levels.

Besides gum problems, diabetes may also cause dry mouth, red or tender gums, bleeding gums, fungal infections, taste impairment, burning tongue, loose teeth, changes in denture fit, and "acetone breath," a distinct telltale mouth odor. That's why dentists are often the first to spot undiagnosed diabetes and/or poor blood-sugar control.

BRUSHING AND FLOSSING

What this means is that you must practice excellent dental hygiene so you won't run into these problems. Using a soft toothbrush (hard ones can scratch the gums) and a fluoride toothpaste, brush your teeth carefully morning and night and after every meal. Don't scrub, but use light downward strokes. Rinse with an antimicrobial mouth rinse.

Then *every night* before going to bed and just after you have brushed your teeth, take some unwaxed dental floss and floss out the plaque that accumulates around each tooth under the gumline in places that the toothbrush doesn't reach. Gently, gently! Ask your dentist or dental hygienist to give you a lesson in the proper way to do this: Wind the ends of the floss around your two forefingers, then *gently* work the taut center section between two teeth. Do not snap it in because you must be careful not to injure your gums. Then, first to the left, then to the right, curving the floss into a C-shape, gently dislodge the plaque from around the gumline of each tooth. When you have done this between all your teeth, rinse out your mouth.

If you are not sure you have done a good job with the flossing, you can buy some special vegetable dye that will show you the places you have missed. It is made for this purpose.

Gum massage is another useful preventive measure because it improves the circulation. After each brushing, take your fingers and gently but firmly give your gums a good rub. Better yet, use a special gum massager with a rubber tip.

See your dentist *at least* every four to six months, both for a good cleaning—it's important that hardened plaque or tartar is removed that often—and to check out your gums. Go to the dentist within the week if you notice any sign of trouble—swelling, soreness, sensitivity, dark spots, white or red patches—anywhere in your mouth. If you have developed periodontal disease, immediate treatment is what you need. Be sure your dentist is thoroughly knowledgeable about gum disease, diabetes, and current methods of treatment and, if necessary, sends you to a periodontist, a dentist who specializes in gum disease.

MORE TOOTH TIPS

• Before you have any dental work done, *including cleaning,* which frequently results in injured gums, you should be "covered" by antibiotics. That means, because you are susceptible to infections, all preventive measures should be taken automatically. You should have three days of antibiotic treatment—the day before, the day of, and the day after the dental work.

· Keep in mind that some drugs, such as Dilantin, can have an adverse effect on your gums.

· If you have periodontal work done on your gums, that doesn't mean you can now forget the flossing and the massage. The problems will return if you don't work hard to prevent them.

· Be sure to get your diabetes under excellent control *before* having any periodontal surgery, so you will have the best chance of fast healing.

· If, because of periodontal work or extractions, you must eat soft or liquid foods for a while, remember that you must still abide by a proper diabetic diet. Liquids are fine, but they may contain calories and perhaps sugar and must be accounted for just as if they were solid foods. If you are confused about substitutions (see Chapter 3), work it out with your doctor or a dietitian *before* you get into trouble.

DIABETES AND YOUR SKIN

For all the same reasons that you tend to get infections more easily than people with normal blood sugar and have a harder time fighting them off, you may discover you have skin problems more often, too. If you do, look to your control. Though the blame for these skin problems may be shared by microvascular changes and sluggish white cells that aren't so quick to attack bacteria and other invaders, remember that high sugar is the real villain, and that skin infections are often the direct result of poorly controlled diabetes. In fact, boils, styes, inflammation around the nails, and other eruptions are often the clues that make a physician suspect diabetes in the first place. Poor control also causes dry, itchy skin, which you may scratch and irritate, issuing an invitation to an invasion of bacteria.

Poor control promotes the appearance of fungus or yeast infections of the vagina in women, of the groin in men, and sometimes of the anus regardless of your gender. Your doctor can prescribe effective medication. Your job is to use it faithfully and get yourself back in good condition. Fungi also make homes in armpits, between fingers and toes, around the nails, and in other moist places. A drug called Lamisil, taken topically or orally, is very effective against fungal infections such as athlete's foot of the feet and hands.

SPOTS AND OTHER PROBLEMS

Fairly common among long-term diabetics is spotted leg syndrome or skin spots. These little brown pockmarks that start out looking like reddish bruises usually appear on the shins where tiny end capillaries have shut down. They don't hurt and they don't get worse, though we know of no way to get rid of them.

A skin condition, necrobiosis lipoidica diabeticorum (NLD), is the special province of diabetics and it, too, is worrisome chiefly for cosmetic reasons. Necrobiosis is the appearance, frequently on the lower legs, of patches of reddish-brown lesions. These become areas of tight, shiny skin like glazed parchment paper that is indented because of a loss of subcutaneous fat just beneath it. Sometimes they are itchy or even painful; or they may crack. The spots are often discolored, but they tend to fade with time although this may take a few years. Some doctors have successfully treated NLD with fine-needle injections of cortisone, though usually no treatment is needed except to prevent injury or infection.

Ulcers, which start out as a skin problem, soon become more than that if the infection deepens and extends into the surrounding tissue. If you discover even the smallest indication of infection, especially on your legs or feet, call your doctor immediately. Prompt treatment to avert big trouble is what you need.

INSULIN ATROPHY AND HYPERTROPHY

A cosmetic problem called lipodystrophy (insulin atrophy and hypertrophy) is, happily, becoming much less common among diabetics today as purer insulins are developed. Insulin atrophy, which appears in areas where insulin injections are given frequently, is a loss of fatty tissue just below the skin, causing large depressions that look scooped out. This can make a person—and usually this happens to young women—most unhappy, although usually the areas eventually fill in again and disappear.

Sometimes insulin injections promote an abnormal buildup of fat, and so you have lumps instead of hollows, or occasionally both. This is called insulin hypertrophy.

To prevent either problem, don't inject into identical sites continually. Rotate your shots so you don't hit the same place more than once a month. Keep a record of your sites to help you do this.

Diabetic blisters (bullosa diabeticorum) are painless raised areas that look like burn blisters. These are quite rare and happen to people whose diabetes is out of control. To get rid of them, attend to your blood sugar. They will disappear in a few weeks.

Small, hard pealike bumps with red halos and an itch are another sign of lack of diabetic control and will disappear when you are in better shape. This condition is known as eruptive xanthomatosis.

EVERYDAY SKIN CARE

If you allow your skin to become dry and chapped—and dry skin is a characteristic of diabetics; in fact, the skin becomes dehydrated when your control is poor—you will not only be inviting bacteria, but you will lower the skin's ability to serve as a barrier to the loss of body water. Don't take too many baths, especially in cold weather. Don't wash too often with soap, and avoid disinfectants or solvents. Try super-fatted soaps. Wear gloves and scarves and warm socks or stockings when you're out in the cold.

To add moisture to your skin and protect it, soak (your whole body or just the dry area) in warm water for several minutes, pat off the excess water, then apply a greasy ointment like petroleum jelly or lanolin, or a good dry-skin cream or lotion.

If you use bath oil, pour the oil in the tub *after* you have soaked yourself for a while. In this way, your skin will first absorb some water which the oil will help to retain. If you put the oil in the water before you have absorbed some moisture into your skin, it will form a barrier to that moisture. Be careful not to slip when you get out!

The same principle applies to moisturizing lotion or cream whose purpose is to seal water in. Wet your skin and pat it almost dry before applying the moisturizer.

THE LINK WITH ALZHEIMER'S DISEASE

Recent studies have linked diabetes with a significantly increased risk of Alzheimer's disease, suggesting that compared with healthy people, those with type 2 diabetes are twice as likely to develop the disease that gradually destroys the brain's ability to function.

According to researchers who presented their findings at the Tenth International Conference on Alzheimer's Disease and Related Disorders in 2006, deposits of amyloid, a type of protein, build up in the brain as well as in the pancreas of diabetics. Others in Germany propose that insulin resistance may cause some of the brain-cell damage. Earlier research, published in 2004 by a medical group at Rush University Medical Center, found that type 2 diabetics had a 65 percent greater risk, along with impairment to memory and problem-solving.

And in a study presented in 2006, Swedish researchers reported that even people with borderline diabetes are more likely than those with normal blood sugar to get Alzheimer's.

What all of this means is that you have one more excellent reason to keep your blood sugar under control. Not every diabetic gets Alzheimer's, and not all Alzheimer's patients are diabetic, but research at Kaiser Permanente in California found that, based on the records of almost 23,000 type 2 diabetics over a period of eight years, the higher the blood sugar, the greater the risk of dementia.

11

RULES FOR SICK DAYS

Just like everybody else, you are going to get sick occasionally. But, unlike everybody else, you will discover your life promptly becomes much more complicated simply because you are a diabetic with an infection. Infections can be more difficult to get rid of and often more severe for you because your defenses may not be the best. Besides, with most illnesses your insulin requirements will rise, sometimes quite dramatically.

All this means that control may be hard to maintain during an illness, so now your objective is not only to recover from the illness but also to avoid acidosis and a trip to the hospital.

If you are on diet alone or diet plus oral agents, remember you are not immune to high blood sugars, acetone, and acidosis when you are sick. You may need temporary shots of insulin to get through, so never neglect your blood tests. Instead of one a day, increase them to three or four. If you normally take insulin, your chief occupation now will be testing your blood and adjusting your dose according to your doctor's instructions. You will undoubtedly need more insulin, maybe two or three times more than usual.

When you are sick, you must live strictly by the rules:

RULE 1:   Stay in close touch with your doctor. The doctor is the person who must make the medical decisions, some major, some minor, when you are sick. Remember the telephone is your friend. If you see a problem evolving call right away. Any doctor would rather hear from you at 6 or 10 P.M. than 2 A.M., but better 2 A.M. than not at all if you are in bad shape.

If you feel your physician doesn't like to be bothered by frequent (not excessive) phone calls or is not providing the guidance you need, find another one. Check with the American Diabetes Association or Juvenile Diabetes Foundation in your area for a recommendation.

RULE 2:   When you are sick, *check your blood at least four times a day,* before each meal and at bedtime. If you are seriously ill, check it every *two* hours, including during the night. Just as you are never too tired to breathe, you are *never* too tired or sick or weak to test yourself. You must know where your blood sugar stands because the test will tell you what to do next.

RULE 3:   When blood sugar is high, the diabetic who takes insulin must compensate with extra insulin, the fast-acting variety. Your doctor will tell you how much to take. It may be 5 units every two hours if your sugar is more than 250, or, if that doesn't do the job, 10 or more units every two hours.

When you get a very high sugar reading, *always test for acetone* (see page 167 for instructions). *The presence of acetone along with high sugar* means you need extra insulin quickly because you may be just one step away from acidosis and a coma. Check for acetone every hour or two so you will know how much trouble you're in. Now you may require even *more* extra fast-acting insulin every two hours until the sugar comes down, according to your doctor's instructions. This is vital if you are going to avoid acidosis.

After you have lowered your blood sugar with increased insulin, it would be wise to set your alarm clock for 3 A.M. Check your blood sugar and eat something if it is low.

However, if your sugar is normal but your acetone is positive, take only your usual dose of insulin. If your sugar is low—under 100 mgs—skip the fast insulin and take your usual dose of insulin. In this case, high acetone means the acetone has not been entirely washed out of the body (it may remain for about twenty-four hours after your sugar has been regulated back to normal); or that your body lacks its primary fuel—sugar—and is burning fat, one of the end products of which is acetone. You now need carbohydrate—juice, bread, cereal, milk, etc.—plus some protein to avoid an insulin reaction now and later in the day and to give your body its normal fuel. Check with your doctor.

Sickness is rarely a major diabetic problem for a person controlled only by diet, but it can be. Even you can develop acidosis if you allow high sugars to persist without taking action. Call your doctor if you have high sugars for more than twenty-four hours. You may require temporary insulin because the stress of illness can raise your insulin requirement far beyond the ability of your pancreas to produce it.

When you take oral agents, your insulin needs will rise during an infection because of the additional release of glucose from the liver. The result may be that the amount of insulin produced by your own pancreas with the help of the oral agent won't be enough to cover the sugar and prevent the end result of acidosis. Your doctor must make the decision as to whether you should take more of the oral agent until your blood sugar drops, or whether you will need insulin injections temporarily. When you have reached or come close to your maximum dosage of oral hypoglycemic agents and continue to have high sugar and produce acetone, you will be instructed to use insulin—either alone or as a supplement to the pills—until your glucose levels are normal once more. Call your doctor, who will probably prescribe 5 to 10 units of fast-acting insulin every two hours until the sugar comes down.

RULE 4: **Always keep fast-acting insulin and a few syringes on hand,** whether or not you normally use them. They may be what you need to counteract high sugar in a hurry. Stash acetone strips in the house, too, along with a glucagon emergency kit (see page 188) just in case of a sudden insulin reaction. All diabetics, even those on oral agents, may come upon a time when for some reason, usually sickness, sugars become very high and acetone lurks. If you have your supplies handy, you can usually take care of the situation yourself and avoid a trip to the emergency room.

RULE 5: *Never* **omit your daily insulin,** *even if you are eating less than usual or not at all,* although you may need a smaller dose. Your diabetes does not disappear just because you can't eat, and your liver continues to manufacture glucose, perhaps much more than usual.

If your blood tests are *normal* or *high, even if you can't eat,* take your usual dose. Then consult with your doctor about an extra amount.

If your sugar is *low* but you cannot eat, take *half* your usual dose. But *never* take nothing or you will end up with acidosis.

Continue to test throughout the day. Don't wait till

tomorrow, hoping you'll wake up cured. You may wake up in the hospital instead.

If you are on oral agents, you can omit your pills when you cannot eat much and your blood sugar is below 100 mgs. Always, of course, check with your doctor.

RULE 6:   Try to eat. Even if you are not hungry or you are nauseated, you can usually find something that will go down and stay there. To prevent acidosis, you need at least 50 to 60 grams of carbohydrate a day. If you can't stick to your usual diet plan, switch over to food that goes down most easily and eat it in smaller amounts spaced throughout the day. If you can't eat normal meals, now is the time for you to eat carbohydrates, so that you get sufficient fuel.

Try toast, crackers, a small amount of regular ginger ale, yogurt, juices, custard, ice cream. Perhaps grapefruit, eggnog, cereal. Your goal should be 10 grams of carbohydrate an hour.

Even though we told you to stay away from apples because they raise your blood sugar too high too quickly, go ahead and eat some applesauce if your sugar is *low* and it is the only food that you can keep down.

Drink plenty of fluids, about 6 to 8 ounces every hour that you're awake. If you can eat, drink sugar-free and caffeine-free liquids.

If liquids are all you can manage, drink your food, remembering that you must have sufficient carbohydrate as well as salt to replace the salt lost by excessive urination. Clear soup, salty broth, tea with sugar, juice, milk, regular (not diet) ginger ale or cola to give you the carbohydrate you need may appeal to you. Take some about every half hour in small amounts.

If you can't eat or drink at all, inform your doctor *im-*

mediately. If you can't reach your doctor, go to an emergency room before you're in really dire straits.

Easy-to-Eat Foods

Applesauce
Bread
Broth, bouillon
Cereal
Coffee
Cottage cheese
Crackers
Custard
Egg
Eggnog
Fruit juices
Ice cream
Ice milk

Jams or jellies, regular
Jell-O, regular
Popsicle
Postum
Sherbet
Soft drinks, regular
Soups
Sugar
Tapioca
Tea
Tomato juice
Vegetable cocktail
Yogurt

RULE 7:   Try to control vomiting as quickly as possible. Three ounces of regular ginger ale or cola every hour often acts as an antiemetic and provides the needed carbohydrate, too. If that doesn't banish the nausea, your doctor can prescribe a suppository or give you an antinausea injection. Tigan suppositories (200 mgs for adults or 100 mgs for children who weigh less than 30 pounds) every eight hours, or Compazine suppositories (up to 25 mgs for adults, 5 mgs for older children, 2.5 mgs for young children) every eight hours are usually effective. A newer drug called Sofran, used by cancer patients to combat nausea after chemotherapy, works well, too. It may be taken by mouth or injection. And if your blood glucose is very low, it is acceptable for you to try Emetrol, a concentrated sugar.

If you can't eat or drink at all or you are continuing to vomit, call your doctor *immediately.* You may need intravenous infusions of saline solution and/or glucose.

Continue to take your usual insulin or oral agent, plus fast-acting insulin every two hours if your sugar is high.

RULE 8:   Control diarrhea as quickly as possible, too, because it can cause the loss of valuable fluids and carbohydrates. Usually a drug such as Lomotil or Imodium works well, but if you have diarrhea and nausea at the same time, you won't be able to keep it down nor can you use suppositories. An intramuscular injection of Compazine, which your doctor can prescribe for nausea, may be the solution. *Call the doctor* for instructions.

RULE 9:   There is no need to stay in bed, but it's important to rest as much as possible. Do not exercise. If you are very sick, it would be advisable to have someone to take care of you.

RULE 10:   If you are taking antibiotics, you will have an increased tendency to get fungal infections—vaginitis, rectal itching, skin infections. When you are given an antibiotic, you should also be given lactobacillus, perhaps acidophilus tablets. Plain yogurt eaten in place of fruit or bread may help prevent an overgrowth of the fungi. Always check the container to make sure it has live cultures.

RULE 11:   Check all medications for sugar. Many cold medicines as well as other drugs are loaded with it and can throw your control off in a hurry. Sudafed and Triaminic syrups, for example, contain 3½ grams of carbohydrate per teaspoon. If you take three teaspoons a day for a cold, you are adding 10½ grams of unwanted simple sugar to your bloodstream. A popular brand of cough syrup contains 2.8 grams per teaspoon, or 11.2

extra grams when you take the recommended 4 tea-spoons a day. Other cold medicines have similar carbo-hydrate contents.

You certainly should not add this much sugar to your body at a time when you are already under the stress of infection and your glucose tolerance is disturbed be-cause of the release of cortisone from your adrenal glands. It is possible, however, to get medications with-out sugar. Cough medicines that are sugar-free include Robitussin SF, Safetussin DM, Sorbutuss, and Diabetic Tussin.

RULE 12:   *Keep a careful record* **of all your test results,** insulin intake, food, and drink. Omit nothing. Write this information down so that you can refer to it when you discuss your situation with your doctor. Include com-ments on how you feel, whether you are vomiting, have diarrhea, a temperature, etc., each time you record your test results.

DIABETES AND SURGERY

Both surgery and physical injuries are an assault on your diabetic control because they stimulate the body's de-fense mechanism to pour out cortisone and adrenaline that increase your blood sugar. So you must double your efforts at these times to maintain good control, making frequent tests and perhaps taking additional insulin.

If you are in good control, you'll have no special problems recovering from surgery and will heal just about as quickly as anyone else. When you expect surgery, bring your sugar into the normal range and keep it there, if you can. Otherwise, you may find that acidosis lurks just around the corner and that you'll heal with difficulty. The best-known anabolic (tissue-building) agent is insulin.

Of course, your doctor is in charge when you are in the hospital and he will make adjustments in your medication to regulate your sugar both during the operative procedure and postoperatively. Your insulin will be increased, or, if you don't normally take it, you may have to go the insulin route temporarily until you are stable once more.

When surgery is scheduled, ask your doctor to make you the first case of the day so your normal routine will be disturbed as little as possible.

If you are on an oral agent, you don't want to take that morning's dose because you won't be eating before the operation and your sugar may fall very low.

If you are on insulin, you will probably be given an intravenous glucose infusion and half of your insulin dose on the morning of the surgery, then insulin as needed after the surgery. I strongly advise that you arrange to be in the care of a qualified diabetologist in addition to the surgeon at this time.

If you're taking Lantus or Levemir insulin, take a smaller dose the night before the surgery—you don't want an insulin reaction on the operating table. And, since you're not going to eat breakfast, don't take any fast-acting insulin in the morning. Take it after the operation, when you're ready to eat.

Even when you are in the hospital, the rules still apply. "They gave it to me" is no excuse for eating so much carbohydrate that your blood sugar will go sky-high. If you are suffering from an infection or the stress of surgery, your blood sugar will tend to run high anyway—don't make it worse by eating the wrong foods (see Chapter 4).

BEWARE OF DRUG INTERACTIONS

If you have an illness that requires you take a drug, be sure your doctor remembers you are a diabetic. If you go to a specialist who does not know your history, give out the information immediately. Not only does your diabetes affect your illness, but the drugs prescribed may affect your diabetes.

For example, oral steroids, such as cortisone, raise insulin requirements. Diabetics on insulin may need a higher dose, and those on diet or oral agents may need to take insulin while on the steroids. Remember that prednisone, Medrol, and dexamethasone are all cortisone drugs.

Dilantin is a major drug used for epilepsy or convulsive disorders. It has the ability to inhibit insulin release, so even people with borderline diabetes can be thrown out of control when they use this drug. It is sometimes prescribed for diabetic neuropathy, but it can be dangerous.

Inderal and other beta blockers, drugs commonly prescribed for angina, headaches, and hypertension, can mask an insulin reaction, too. When blood sugar is low, the adrenal glands secrete adrenaline, which releases sugar from the liver. A rapid heartbeat, sweating, and other symptoms usually alert you to the fact that you are becoming hypoglycemic, but Inderal blocks this effect so that you may not be aware of your precarious situation.

Other drugs affect the action of oral agents, too, enhancing their effectiveness and sometimes producing hypoglycemic reactions. These include: some antidepressants, antipsychotics, beta blockers, niacin, epilepsy drugs, thiazide diuretics, and a number of other medications. Certain antibiotics, such as Biaxin, Levaquin, and Tequin, can also raise blood-sugar levels precipitously.

And there's more to worry about: The effect of barbiturates, sedatives, and hypnotics can be greatly prolonged when they are taken together with oral antidiabetic agents. And the effect of the oral agents may be prolonged as well, giving you another way to have reactions.

Don't take any chances. Before you take a new drug, remind your doctor and your pharmacist that you are a diabetic on insulin or oral agents—they may not think of it—and always ask if a new drug might have an effect on your sugar control.

12

WATCHING YOUR FEET

When you are a diabetic, you hear a lot about taking good care of your feet. It may seem like a minor issue, but it's extremely important that you follow all the rules about foot care if you want to avoid some very unpleasant problems in the future. Any injuries or infections of the feet and ankles and even lower legs are potentially very dangerous to the diabetic. They can lead to serious complications that can be treated only by drastic surgery, which you don't even want to think about. The most common reason for the amputation of feet and legs is long-term diabetes, so the big word now is *prevention*. Don't let anything get started. And if it should, go *immediately* to your doctor.

Foot sores are the most common reason for hospitalization for diabetics. About a quarter of all people with diabetes, and half of the diabetics over sixty-five, develop them. About half of the ulcers become infected and, of these, 20 percent require surgery. The good news is that most of them are preventable. So listen carefully to the advice you're about to read.

A diabetic, especially if control has been poor for a number of years, tends to have poor circulation in the legs and feet. This is particularly true for older people. The small arteries become narrower and cannot carry the optimum amounts of blood, oxygen, and infection-fighting white cells to these extremities. That makes diabetics particularly susceptible to injuries, calluses, and infections such as carbuncles, boils, and athlete's foot, which can become serious problems *very* quickly. It also tends to reduce sweat production, which can lead to dry skin that cracks and becomes infected more easily.

Sometimes the nerve endings, as well as the circulation, are affected. Diabetics often have neuropathy—damage to the small sensory nerves—and that means you may not have the feeling in your feet that you once had. You can cut yourself, wear shoes that rub, step on sharp objects, or burn yourself and never realize it. You can get athlete's foot or other infections without knowing it. Meanwhile, the wound or infection can rapidly turn into a major problem. For a nondiabetic, a little cut, a rub, a blister, a fungus may be only an annoyance. For a diabetic, any foot injury that's neglected can lead to an ulcer. This could be the start of deep trouble, so you can't let it go, even for a few days.

That's why, though you may find it a nuisance, you must consciously pay attention to your feet every single day. Actually it's easy and takes only a few minutes, and it wouldn't be a bad idea if everyone did the same thing. Feet are rarely anyone's favorite part of the body and are usually totally ignored and maltreated until they start causing some discomfort. But you can't afford to ignore yours—you *must* head off any problems before they begin if you possibly can.

You have to abide by a list of simple rules of hygiene, remember a number of things you should and should not do, make periodic appointments with a reputable podiatrist, and, most important, waste no time in checking with your podiatrist and/or your doctor if you notice the slightest sign of a problem, even a small discoloration. Never assume that whatever it is will just clear

up on its own. It might, but it might not. Never treat
your feet yourself except under the direction of your
doctor. Never assume anything is too minor to worry
about. Always remember *you must not wait* until you
feel pain to become concerned—you may not feel a
thing and yet be brewing serious problems. Don't take
any chances.

BE SURE YOU GET A THOROUGH EXAMINATION

Whenever you see your doctor, whether for a routine
exam or because something seems amiss, insist on a
close inspection of your feet and legs. You should remove your shoes and socks so the doctor can check the
pulses of your feet and the integrity of your skin, look
for calluses and corns and other problems, compare one
foot against the other, and screen you for neuropathy.

All of these procedures are essential if you are going
to avoid serious foot problems. To test for a dangerous
decline in sensation that can signal nerve damage and
lead to neuropathic ulcers, the doctor may use a simple
inexpensive monofilament device, a special brush with a
single nylon bristle. The brush is pressed against various
spots on the feet and lower legs to gauge the feeling in
these areas. It has been estimated that annual testing for
lost sensation could prevent 80 to 90 percent of all foot
amputations caused by these problems.

In addition, the physician should check the blood
flow in your feet and legs with a Doppler meter because
you also have a tendency to have compromised blood
circulation—peripheral arterial disease (PAD)—in your
lower extremities that can lead to serious complications.
Blood pressure in the ankles should also be checked. If it

is significantly lower than the blood pressure in your arms, PAD may be narrowing the arteries in your legs.

A recent study has found that checking the skin temperature on the bottom of your feet with a special hand-held infrared thermometer every day is another good way to head off problems. If either foot is warmer than 90 degrees, or if one foot is 4 degrees warmer than the other, consider it an early warning sign that an ulcer may be developing and you should see your doctor as soon as you can.

Under development is yet another way to detect changes in the skin and catch problems before it is too late. It is called medical hyperspectral imaging and it measures the oxygen levels of the feet. Low levels mean you need to pay especially close attention to your feet, checking regularly for small injuries that may progress to big problems.

If you have an ulcer, you will require an X-ray and/or a white-blood-cell scan to look for bone damage or joint degeneration and tests to rule out infection. Ask your doctor about Regranex (becaplermin), a topical gel that may help heal the injuries by stimulating new tissue growth.

EVERYDAY FOOT CARE

WASHING

Wash your feet every day. Yes, every day. They must be kept clean. This does not mean soaking them, not a wise practice for diabetics. In fact, it is dangerous and actually encourages infection by softening the skin so much that it may break easily and provide a home for bacteria and fungi.

Because your skin is probably very dry, use a nonalkaline soap. (If you're not sure which brands are nonalkaline, ask your druggist for one. It will not require a prescription.) Be especially careful to avoid deodorant soaps, which are particularly drying.

Be sure the water is only warm (below 92° F.), *never hot*. If you have a loss of pain perception, common in many diabetics, you may not notice the water is too hot if you carelessly dip your feet in without testing it first. Don't test with your toe. Use your hand or your elbow. Or use a thermometer. One thing you must not have is burned feet.

Now take a soft towel and carefully dry your feet. Do not rub between your toes, because the skin here is thin and delicate, but pat off the moisture to avoid irritation.

EXAMINING

This is the moment to take a close look at every square millimeter of your feet and lower legs. Every day. If your eyesight isn't good or you have trouble bending over that far, enlist someone else to do this. If you can't see the bottoms of your feet, use a mirror or ask your significant other to do it for you. We'll say it again: If you see any broken skin, peeling, redness, irritation, blisters, bruises, swelling, *anything* that even vaguely strikes you as unusual, don't treat it yourself and don't waste a moment. Go immediately to your podiatrist or physician.

By the way, every diabetic should have a good podiatrist, a specialist in foot care. Podiatrists are frequently much more knowledgeable about foot and leg problems than most physicians.

SKIN CARE

After you have examined your feet closely, sprinkle some baby powder between your toes. Then gently rub a skin-softening lotion or cream on your feet and legs to counteract the dryness, except between your toes, where you do not want moisture. Avoid any lotions that contain medication or alcohol.

GO TO YOUR PODIATRIST

For most diabetics, it is an excellent idea to go to a podiatrist as often as necessary to have your toenails trimmed. It is much better than doing it yourself. That's because a small slip of the scissors can be the start of trouble. Especially if your toenails are thick—as they often are in older people—it is best for an expert to do the job. Besides, your visit will be an opportunity for this expert to check out your feet to be sure all is well. You will have a chance to ask questions and get advice, eliminating vague worries from your mind and forestalling any ill-advised self-treatment.

If you are going to do the pedicuring yourself at any time, keep the following rules in mind. Use manicuring scissors with blunt rounded tips, the kind used for cutting babies' nails. Cut your nails after a bath so they will be soft. Trim them *straight across,* even with the ends of your toes. If they are too long, you will have pressure on the nail bed; if they are too short, they will not protect your toes as they are intended to do and may expose the fragile skin beneath them.

Never cut cuticles or skin. Don't cut in at the corners, because you will not only be in danger of cutting into the skin but you will also invite ingrown toenails. Don't use a nail file to keep your toenails in shape because you may unwittingly file your skin and irritate it. But you should use an emery board with a light touch to smooth down any rough edges.

If someone else does this job for you, be sure that person knows how to do it the right way. Give him/her this chapter to read.

BEWARE OF PEDICURES

Pedicures can be bad news for diabetics. If you have any breaks in your skin and the tools the operator uses aren't sterilized between clients, you could be infected with the last customer's germs. If your calluses or cuticles are trimmed too aggressively, you could end up with small nicks and cuts that can provide the perfect environment for an infection. Better to skip the beauty treatment unless you're absolutely sure that the premises and the pedicurist follow the rules of good hygiene.

EVEN MORE ADVICE

Now you may be thinking that all these rules about your feet are excessive, but we are going to add more anyway. If you want to stay in good shape, with two strong healthy feet holding you up for the rest of your life, don't skip to the next chapter but keep reading.

CHECK OUT YOUR FOOTWEAR

Change your socks every day, more often if they get wet or your feet sweat a lot. If they don't fit perfectly, give them away. Your socks must not be too large or too small. They must not form wrinkles in your shoes. They must not have prominent seams; in fact, there are special seamless socks made for diabetics. They must not have holes. They must not be mended. Stretch socks or hosiery are not a good idea for you because they may re-strict circulation or put pressure on your toes. Never wear socks or stockings with elasticized tops for the same reason. Furthermore, garters are out. Cotton or wool socks are the best choices because they are more absorbent than the synthetic fibers. When hiking, wear lightweight socks under regular-weight socks.

Never, never wear shoes that don't fit perfectly and comfortably. Each foot has 26 bones and 78 joints that must be well treated. Be sure there is enough room to ac-commodate all your toes in their natural positions, and that the heel is snug enough not to slide up and down. Buy shoes in the afternoon, when your feet are the largest, and always have your feet measured standing, not sitting. Feet tend to get larger as you get older, so do not assume you wear the same size without checking. Choose shoes made of leather, not plastic, to allow more air circulation. If you are an animal rights supporter who won't wear leather, find fabric shoes or plastic shoes with pores or airholes.

If your sensory perception is not too good, you may not feel rubbing, so be sure to watch for it every time you take off your shoes and during your daily ablutions. Don't wear open toes—closed toes give much more pro-tection. Break in new shoes gradually by wearing them around the house and then on short jaunts.

Get in the habit of feeling the insides of your shoes be-fore you put them on, to be sure there aren't any pro-truding nails, bumps, torn linings, or rough spots that may be hazards.

If you can't find shoes that fit right, consult with your podiatrist, who may have a solution for you.

Going barefoot, even in the house, is not for you. The minute you step out of bed in the morning, put on a pair of slippers or shoes. Wear swim shoes or sneakers on the beach. Don't take a chance on stubbing your toe, getting a splinter, stepping on a piece of glass or a sharp shell, burning your feet on hot sand or cement.

SOME IMPORTANT DON'TS

• Don't use medications or chemicals on your feet unless prescribed by your doctor (again be sure the doctor remembers you are diabetic). This includes over-the-counter foot remedies. Powerful medications, such as iodine, or medicated materials such as corn plasters, can destroy tissue or cause burns to delicate skin. A good rule is: If you can't put it on your face, don't put it on your feet. Tinted medicines, Mercurochrome, for example, are taboo, too, because they can camouflage inflammation.

• Don't try bathroom surgery with scissors, razors, or even pumice stones or corn pads. If you develop a corn or a callus—which you shouldn't because you've thrown out your ill-fitting shoes—leave it alone! Let your podiatrist treat it. If you have poor weight distribution, which may be causing the corns or calluses, this specialist may make a mold for you to wear in your shoe to correct the problem. Do not mess with blisters either. Never open them.

• Don't use heat on your feet. Never put your feet in hot water. Remember to test the bathwater with your hand or elbow. Stay out of saunas, steam rooms, whirlpool baths—most of them are too hot for your feet. Apply lots of sunscreen lotion when you are out in the sun—don't let your feet get sunburned. *Never* use hot-water bottles or heating pads.

• Don't let your feet get too chilled, either. Because your blood vessels are probably narrower and more constricted when you have diabetes, it's easier for you to get frostbite. Invest in warm (but smooth) socks and roomy boots for cold weather. But don't wear boots indoors all day, because they can impede your circulation and, because they are warm, make your feet sweat and become susceptible to bacteria.

• Don't use adhesive tape. It can irritate the skin or even pull some skin away when you take it off. Instead, use "ouchless" bandages or tape.

• Don't stay in bed for more than a day without protecting your heels with an "egg-crate" pad under your feet and special heel pads to shield them from rubbing. This is especially important when you are hospitalized because ulcers can develop very quickly on diabetic feet. Insist on these protections *on day one* of your stay. Do not wait for a problem to develop before taking action.

• Don't smoke. Just one cigarette will constrict your peripheral blood vessels to an astonishing degree. Since yours are probably already narrower than normal, smoking will only compound the situation.

That is a lot of nevers and don'ts, but all must be heeded.

GOT A PROBLEM?

Do not waste a second if you notice a lesion on a foot or a leg. Get yourself to your doctor that very day because lesions must be treated aggressively and quickly with oral or topical antibiotics if they are not to become serious problems. If your physician is not experienced in dealing with diabetic ulcers, ask for a referral.

GET ENOUGH EXERCISE

You need some kind of exercise every day because it will improve your circulation and encourage collateral vascular development. When your feet and the rest of you are in good condition, there is no exercise you can't do—from tennis to running to ice hockey. Nonathletes can move their blood around most efficiently by swimming or walking briskly at least a half hour every day.

CAUTION: if you have a foot or lower leg injury or infection, this is not the time for exercise. Even if it doesn't hurt, walking on injuries can damage them further.

13

MANAGING A DIABETIC PREGNANCY

Can I have a baby? Will I have problems conceiving? Will the baby be normal? How risky is pregnancy for me? How will it affect my diabetes? Will the baby be diabetic? These are questions of immense importance to young women with diabetes. Happily, the answers today are astonishingly positive. Not many years ago, a diabetic woman conceived with difficulty and embarked on a hazardous trip when she became pregnant, with a good chance of losing her baby on the way and endangering her own health.

But today, the vast majority of diabetic women can have healthy babies, with only a slightly higher than normal statistical chance of miscarriage, congenital anomalies, and stillbirths, even in the presence of some serious diabetic complications. According to the Joslin Clinic, the fetal survival rate of diabetic pregnancies is now about 97 percent, while the rate for nondiabetics is 98 or 99 percent. That is a remarkably small difference. And maternal deaths today are almost nonexistent.

Managing a diabetic pregnancy, however, requires excellent medical care, as well as complete cooperation on your part. This venture demands total dedication and motivation, hard work, time, and attention. Besides, a diabetic pregnancy can be expensive. You may need the expert medical care of a whole team of specialists, many office visits, perhaps a number of hospitalizations, so-phisticated laboratory tests, possibly a cesarean delivery.

For a happy outcome to a diabetic pregnancy, ex-tremely tight blood-sugar control is the key. What we look for is blood sugar under 100 mgs percent before breakfast and less than 120 mgs two hours after eating. This is not so easy for an insulin-dependent woman, though it can definitely be achieved if you work at it. If you are controlled by diet alone, it is all much simpler. You may get along well simply by watching what you eat, paying strict attention to your sugar levels, and stay-ing in close touch with your obstetrician and internist. Or you may need insulin temporarily because you don't produce enough yourself to satisfy the huge demands of a pregnancy.

If you are normally controlled by diet and oral hypo-glycemic agents, you must now switch to insulin until after the baby is born. This is because the oral agents will not only stimulate your pancreas but the baby's as well. Because it is not yet known whether the oral drugs cross over into breast milk, it is also recommended—if you are going to breast-feed—that you continue on in-sulin until the baby is weaned if strict diet does not give you sufficient control. Glucose also crosses over into the baby's bloodstream, but insulin does not. Instead the baby makes his own.

PLAN AHEAD

Ideally, you should have your babies early in life. And you should plan ahead, decide when to conceive, get yourself into the best possible physical shape before you begin your pregnancy, because the first few weeks of life are the times when your baby's organs are formed. This means your diabetes is under excellent control, you are not overweight, and you have resolved any important medical problems before you start off. You have had your blood pressure, heart, kidneys, nerves, and eyes checked. Some doctors even recommend, as a prelude to pregnancy, that a diabetic woman check into the hospital for at least a few days for evaluation and glucose regulation. If you followed the earlier rules this should not be necessary. At least one study has demonstrated that the babies of women with the lowest hemoglobin A1c, blood-sugar levels measured over two or three months, have the fewest abnormalities.

Once you are pregnant, don't waste a moment starting your prenatal care. Your insulin requirements will change radically and quickly. Good diabetic control—whether or not you take insulin—is particularly important during the first two months, the time when much of the baby's initial development occurs.

A team of medical experts will manage your pregnancy—an obstetrician, a diabetologist (a physician who is a diabetic specialist), perhaps a dietitian, laboratory technicians, later a pediatrician who specializes in perinatology. You will probably visit the obstetrician every week or two until about the thirtieth week, then more often after that. You may consult with the dietitian now and then and see your diabetic specialist twice a month. There are also high-risk obstetricians and neonatologists who specialize in diabetic pregnancies.

CONCEIVING YOUR BABY

If you are healthy, you can get pregnant just as easily as anyone else. Diabetes does not interfere with your fertility when you are well controlled, although you may lose some reproductive years for two reasons. Girls diagnosed with type 1 diabetes before the age of ten may have a delayed menarche (first menstrual period) and an increased incidence of menstrual irregularities, in most cases longer cycles and fewer periods than other women. To complicate matters, diabetic women—both type 1 and type 2—usually have an earlier menopause. Estimates are that 60 percent have menopause before age forty-seven, at an average age of forty-two. The average age for other women is close to fifty.

A diabetic husband, however, may be a source of conception difficulties (see Chapter 14).

IF YOUR HUSBAND IS DIABETIC

Having a diabetic husband will not affect your pregnancy at all, whether or not you are diabetic yourself.

CHOOSING YOUR OBSTETRICIAN

Unfortunately, many good obstetricians do not have expert knowledge of the special problems of diabetic pregnancies. Nor do many hospitals have the facilities and laboratories you may need. Especially if you take insulin, it is essential that you check out the obstetricians and hospitals in your area. Much depends on the kind of medical care you will receive.

If you are already seeing a diabetologist, this doctor will know where to refer you. If you are not going to a diabetologist, we suggest you find one now, or at least an internist who has been recommended by your local Juvenile Diabetes Foundation or American Diabetes Association affiliate. You will need the services of this doctor along with those of the obstetrician. He/she must be available to you night and day—as this person should be even when you aren't pregnant.

The diabetic organizations will also recommend obstetricians, as well as the best hospital for you. Or you can call the department of obstetrics and gynecology at the nearest large hospital or medical school for the names of doctors with special expertise in diabetic pregnancies. Do not, unless you have no choice and no chance of moving, pick an obstetrician simply because your next-door neighbor likes him. You require a person who is an expert.

WHAT KIND OF DIABETIC ARE YOU?

Pregnant diabetic women have been classified into eight groups, so potential problems may be more easily predicted. The classifications, originated by Dr. Priscilla White of the Joslin Clinic, range from those with the mildest diabetic indications to those with the most serious complications. Obviously, women who fit in the early categories usually have the fewest difficulties during pregnancy because their diabetes has had less effect on their bodies' ability to go through the incredibly complicated process of creating a baby.

Here are the classes of pregnant diabetic women:

Class A: Gestational diabetics, women who have abnormal glucose tolerance during pregnancy only. For them, the condition is transient. They have no symptoms and diet is usually the only treatment they require.

Class B: Women whose diabetes began after age twenty and have had it less than ten years. They have no evidence of kidney or eye disease.

Class C: Women who have been diabetic for ten to

twenty years, and were diagnosed between the ages of ten to nineteen. Again, no evidence of serious complications.

Class D: Women who were diagnosed before age ten and have had diabetes over twenty years. They have early retinopathy and/or some kidney damage, calcified blood vessels of the legs, or hypertension.

Class R: Women who have proliferative retinopathy or vitreous hemorrhage.

Class F: Women who have developed neuropathy and/or proteinuria over 500 mgs per day.

Class RF: Women with arteriosclerotic heart disease.

Class T: Women who have had a renal transplantation.

ALL ABOUT GESTATIONAL DIABETES

Sometimes women who have never before shown signs of diabetes develop abnormal glucose tolerance for the first time during a pregnancy, especially if they are 20 percent or more over their ideal weight. The rate of this kind of diabetes increased 35 percent during the 1990s, most noticeably among younger obese women, according to Kaiser Permanente's division of research in California. They are called gestational diabetics, and unless their diabetes preexisted and is only now being discovered, they can expect to lose the disease as soon as the baby is born, although it is likely that it will return in future pregnancies.

Affecting 4 percent (about 136,000) of pregnant American women a year, gestational diabetes occurs when a woman cannot produce the tremendous amount of insulin required by pregnancy. This type of diabetes triggers serious problems. It increases the chances of premature birth, and it triples the risk of an abnormally large baby, along with a greatly increased chance of the need for a cesarean section. It typically afflicts women who are overweight, who had it in a previous pregnancy, and who have a family history of type 2 diabetes.

It's important to remember that this temporary abnormality, which usually shows up around the 24th to 28th week of pregnancy, is a sign that diabetes may occur sometime later in life, and additional pregnancies may add to the strain on an already vulnerable pancreas. Among women who deliver babies weighing more than nine pounds, about 25 percent develop the disease within five years, and 60 percent within twelve years. Each 10 pounds gained after a diabetic pregnancy also increases the risk. The baby's chance of developing diabetes later in life is tripled, which is more reason to keep him at a healthy weight.

If you are diagnosed with this transient condition, you must start treatment immediately to bring your blood-sugar levels down to normal. And here's the good news. If you seek treatment, you will probably have a normal-size baby and no problems with delivery. In most cases, it involves nothing more than a healthy diet and regular exercise. If you are among the minority who don't respond well enough to these lifestyle changes, you'll need insulin temporarily until the baby is born. Again, don't worry about the insulin affecting the baby, as it does not cross the placenta.

WHAT IS A PREDIABETIC?

A prediabetic is someone who has higher-than-normal blood sugar and is probably going to become diabetic, and many pregnant women fit into this group. Pregnancy puts a stress on the pancreas, and if your pancreas has inherited a tendency to diabetes, this may be the time when it will become apparent, the more likely the more pregnancies you have. If you are overweight, remember that every 20 percent of excess weight increases your chances even more.

Because pregnancy is such a common time for diabetes to show up, your obstetrician should perform a routine urinalysis at every visit. Sugar in the urine, however, doesn't have to mean you are diabetic. During any pregnancy, the flow of blood to the kidneys increases and sugar absorption decreases, resulting in more spilled sugar than normal.

But increased glucose in the urine must always be investigated. If you are spilling more sugar than normal, your obstetrician will check for sugar in the blood by giving you an isolated glucose tolerance test using 50 grams of sugar. If after one hour you show a blood-glucose level of more than 130 mgs percent, then you will now require a formal glucose tolerance test (see page 25) to confirm a diagnosis of gestational diabetes.

WHAT IS DIFFERENT ABOUT A DIABETIC PREGNANCY?

Unless you have had diabetes for many years, have serious complications, or are in poor diabetic control, you do not have a higher chance of miscarriage than any other woman. And you will probably carry your baby to term, or close to it. If your diabetes is more severe, your baby may be delivered early.

Because good control is the road to a happy and successful outcome, constant vigilance is essential. Along with all those scheduled visits to your doctors, you must test your blood for sugar four times a day, adjusting your medication accordingly.

Though the insulin you take does not cross the placenta to the fetus, blood sugar does. This means that when your blood sugar goes up, so does the baby's. This stimulates the immature pancreas to produce too much insulin. Excessive insulin promotes the deposition of fat, and so, even if you are a mild diabetic, your baby is likely to be quite large. This fact alone may mean you will need a cesarean delivery. With excellent control, you can probably keep your baby down to a more normal size, however, and have a normal-term delivery.

Severe diabetics, on the other hand, sometimes have very small babies, because vascular complications involving the placenta may restrict the fetal blood supply and therefore the nourishment the fetus receives.

A frequent problem in diabetic pregnancy is hydramnios, an excessive amount of amniotic fluid, which can make you very uncomfortable and perhaps cause premature labor. At the first sign of hydramnios, you will probably be instructed to stay in bed to reduce the volume of fluid.

Other possible special problems include kidney and vascular complications as a result of damage caused by long-term diabetes; and toxemia, a condition that is becoming much less prevalent as knowledge of the value of good control increases. Because in pregnancy there is a greater tendency toward urinary infections, your urine should be checked regularly.

HOW PREGNANCY AFFECTS YOUR DIABETES

Because carrying a baby is a severe stress on your pancreas, your need for insulin will skyrocket during your pregnancy, doubling or even tripling. But in the first trimester (up to 13 weeks), your need will probably *drop,* and you will have to keep adjusting your dose downward (with the help of your doctor) while watching out for hypoglycemic reactions.

Reactions during these early weeks are very common and may occur without any warning, though medical consensus is that they won't hurt the baby. Don't make a move without your emergency sugar, be sure other people know how to handle possible reactions by giving you sugar or glucagon injections if you can't take it by mouth, and make certain your doctor is always available for consultation.

The dip in insulin need is probably due to the large amount of glucose the developing fetus and placenta are using, along with the effect of other hormonal changes, and perhaps morning sickness. You may not be eating (or keeping down) as much food as you usually do. Try to eat foods that appeal to you, space them out in small amounts throughout the day. This phase will soon pass and many women don't experience it at all. If necessary, your doctor may prescribe an antinausea drug. Or, when you can't keep anything down, drink three ounces of *regular* ginger ale every three hours until the nausea passes. Do not drink diet ginger ale. You will need the sugar in a regular soda. Besides, it is probably best to avoid unnecessary chemicals during pregnancy.

After the first two or three months, there is another big change. Now your insulin requirements start rising sharply and you must keep increasing your dose. Along with insulin shock, which remains a distinct possibility, you must be on the alert for the other extreme—acidosis. This, too, can come on very quickly now, and is a much more serious situation. If your tests are poor, if you have an infection, or if you are nauseated, very thirsty, breathless, or have any of the other symptoms of high sugar, check with your doctor immediately. Untreated, acidosis can be harmful to your baby.

Toward the end, around your eighth month, your insulin needs will probably stop rising and will level off.

After the baby is born, they will make another dramatic drop. You may not require any insulin for a few days, or much less than your usual dose. Then gradually, well within six weeks, you will return to your prepregnancy dose. In the meantime, watch out for reactions.

SPLIT DOSES ARE BEST

Pregnant diabetics who require insulin do best with split doses, usually taking both fast-acting and Intermediate-acting insulin before breakfast and again before dinner. The fast-acting insulin takes care of breakfast and dinner; the Intermediate insulin takes care of lunch and the night, so that all bases are covered. In addition, you may need more shots if your sugar is high at any time during the day. You must respond to the information you get from your four daily blood-sugar tests.

If, however, you are taking one of the extra-long-acting insulins Lantus or Detemir at night (and perhaps in the morning) plus a shot of fast-acting insulin before each meal, you need not change your schedule. Take them just the way you always have, with, of course, the approval of your doctor.

If you never took insulin before your pregnancy, you probably won't need it after it's over. You may now return to your simple diet control or diet combined with oral agents. To return to oral agents, your doctor will probably ask you to take your prepregnancy dose and, if you have high sugar, to cover it with insulin before dinner and at bedtime. In a few days, you will know what your correct oral agent dose should be. If you are breast-feeding, do not go back to the pills until the baby is weaned.

WHAT IS GOOD CONTROL NOW?

Though other numbers may be tolerated when you are not pregnant, good control at this time translates to a blood-sugar level of *no lower than* 70 mgs, and *no higher than* 100 mgs fasting and 120 mgs two hours after a meal. This takes careful attention to your diet, and constant adjustments of your insulin if you require it. It also requires blood tests four times a day. It's surprising how many women, after playing fast and loose with their diabetes for years, become model patients when they are carrying a baby. Their concern for the baby makes them change their lifestyles radically, we hope forever.

You must check your blood four times a day, before breakfast, lunch, and bedtime, being sure to be accurate. Just to be safe, however, test for acetone every morning and whenever your sugar reads over 250 mg/dl. Acidosis is always a distinct possibility during pregnancy, and it may happen very quickly, so you must be constantly on the alert.

USING THE INSULIN PUMP

In the few instances when a pregnant woman's diabetes continues to soar out of control despite her best efforts, doctors sometimes recommend an insulin pump (see page 155). This is a gadget worn around the waist. It infuses a few units of insulin per hour through a subcutaneous catheter and gives more before each meal, simulating the normal pancreatic output. Again, the goal is to maintain fasting sugar below 100 mgs and two hours after a meal no more than 120 mgs percent. Carefully attended, the pump can obviously provide excellent diabetic control.

EATING FOR TWO

We haven't talked about total calories before, but now that you are pregnant, this becomes necessary. Most pregnant women require from 1,800 to 2,000 calories of food a day, but the amount that is right for you must be decided together with your doctor or a dietitian. Be sure to eat everything on your meal plan and eat it *on time*. When you strive to maintain the excellent blood-sugar control that is so important now, insulin reactions (if you are insulin-dependent) are always a possibility, even after the first trimester.

When you are pregnant, you will need more protein than at other times. Include two to five glasses of milk (skim or regular) during the day. You may also increase your usual meat portion at dinner.

Space your food throughout the day so your blood sugar doesn't rise and fall sharply. Your developing baby needs a constant supply of nutrients.

Take a daily multivitamin tablet that includes folic acid.

WILL THE BABY BE HEALTHY?

If you're in good control and the baby is mature, your child has just about as good a chance of entering the world in as good a condition as any other infant. The baby will not be born diabetic. In fact, there is a likelihood of hypoglycemia—low blood sugar—for a few hours or days after birth. While still in the uterus, the fetus was exposed to your blood sugar and the tiny pancreas responded by producing large amounts of insulin. A short period of time is needed now to settle down to normal. The pediatrician will have blood tests made to see if the baby requires supplements of sugar given by bottle or intravenously to compensate for the excessive insulin still being turned out.

Other possible results of the baby's long exposure to high sugar include low blood calcium and high blood bilirubin (which causes jaundice), neither of which is reason for serious concern today. Your pediatrician will be alerted to these complications and can correct them. Jaundice rarely needs more than a few days' exposure to ultraviolet lights, and low calcium is treated with intravenous calcium infusions. Babies born to diabetic mothers are usually kept in the nursery's intensive-care unit for a few days for close observation and, if necessary, treatment. Premature babies, of course, may require much longer hospital stays and special care by a team of neonatal specialists, but most infants are ready to go home with their mothers.

The almost certain likelihood of a healthy baby and an uncomplicated delivery applies to diabetic women who keep their diabetes under excellent control during their pregnancies. The rate of problems rises precipitously among women who are poorly controlled.

WILL THE BABY BE DIABETIC?

Your baby will not be born diabetic. But, with a diabetic parent, there is a 1 percent chance your child will develop diabetes before the age of twenty and a 12 percent chance of developing it in his lifetime. Those are not overwhelming odds when you consider that 6 percent of the general population has the very same risk. With two type 2 diabetic parents, however, the chances rise to about 50 percent sometime in a life span.

By the way, a father who gets type 1 diabetes before the age of fifteen has a much greater chance of passing this disease along to a child than does a mother with type 1. But type 2 is different. Here the mother is the one who is more likely to have a child who develops type 2 diabetes.

DO DIABETIC COMPLICATIONS GET WORSE DURING A PREGNANCY?

They could, especially if you do not maintain excellent control. On the other hand, they may improve. One study of a group of pregnant women with retinopathy reported that a third of the women were found to have improved by the time of delivery, a third stayed the same, and a third got worse. If your eyes happen to get worse, they can be treated at the onset to forestall further problems (see Chapter 10). It has been found, moreover, that eyes that become worse during pregnancy usually go back to their former condition afterward.

Although kidney problems may increase during a pregnancy, women with mild kidney disease usually return to their prepregnant situation after their babies are born. However, according to a recent study, for women with moderate-to-severe kidney disease, there is a 45 percent chance that pregnancy will make it worse. In the meantime, kidney problems can make the pregnancy harder to manage.

TIMING YOUR BABY'S ARRIVAL

Once it was true that many babies of diabetic mothers died in the last few weeks of pregnancy, and so it became customary to deliver the babies long before their due date. This led to problems. Because diabetic women sometimes have irregular periods, it wasn't easy to pinpoint the correct delivery time, and the babies were frequently brought into the world, usually by cesarean, before they were ready and suffered from all the problems associated with prematurity.

Today, however, sophisticated tests are available in most medical centers for measuring both fetal health and maturity. Every diabetic woman must be closely monitored, especially as she nears her due date, but Class A and Class B diabetics who do not have complications can often go all the way to term and deliver their babies in the usual fashion.

More severe diabetics are delivered earlier, usually by the 38th or 40th week, but in most of these cases only after it has been determined that their babies are mature enough for this world. In these cases, labor is induced or a cesarean section is performed.

Many obstetricians put their diabetic patients into the hospital for their last two or three weeks, so they can be closely watched. Often, this is the best place to be.

Nonstress testing—monitoring contractions and the baby's heart rate—should start at the 28th week of the pregnancy and will also help the doctor decide when the baby should be delivered.

TESTING FOR MATURITY

Not many babies of diabetic mothers are delivered too early today, because now there are standard tests available at all large hospitals or in laboratories to determine whether they are mature enough to be born. The major problem of premature babies is respiratory distress syndrome (RDS), which means that the tiny lungs are not yet prepared to breathe air efficiently.

To predict lung maturity, amniotic fluid can be tested for the presence of a substance called phosphodidyl glycerate. If enough of this substance is present, the baby's lungs are considered developed enough for delivery. Biophysical profiles (ultrasound) that monitor the rate of the baby's growth are another way that maturity can be estimated.

Sometimes the obstetrician will decide it is best to deliver your baby even though the lungs are not fully mature. In this case you may be given a few doses of corticosteroids, which usually stimulate the production of enough phosphodidyl glycerate within only 24 hours to ensure a safe delivery.

CAN YOU BREAST-FEED YOUR BABY?

Being a diabetic mother doesn't affect your ability to breast-feed, except that getting started may be a little more difficult if you are separated from your baby for very long after the birth. But even if you can't start immediately, it is quite possible to express your milk manually or with a pump so you will continue to produce milk until you need it.

The baby will not be affected by the insulin you take, and won't have insulin reactions. You will probably require less insulin while you are breast-feeding because the baby is consuming some of your glucose supply in the milk, so be alert to your own possible reactions and make adjustments in your dosage if your sugar tends to fall very low.

Because breast-feeding can cause rapid drops in glucose levels, be sure to have a carbohydrate snack before each nursing session.

You must also adjust your diet, adding about 600 to 900 calories a day to compensate for the amount you are expending. Extra milk is an excellent way to get those calories.

Remember that you must not take oral agents while you are breast-feeding. If diet isn't doing the job of controlling your blood sugar, you must take insulin temporarily.

COW'S MILK OR BREAST MILK?

It was once thought that babies who drink cow's milk have an increased risk of developing diabetes. But not to worry. Research at the University of Colorado School of Medicine in Denver found that early exposure to cow's milk is not associated with beta-cell autoimmunity, an early predictor of type 1 diabetes.

On the other hand, extended breast-feeding seems to lower the risk of type 2 diabetes for the mother. Researchers at Harvard Medical School found that for each year a woman breast-feeds, she reduces her risk by 15 percent.

14

SEX AND THE DIABETIC

Does being diabetic affect your sex life? It can, especially if you are a man. It is estimated that about half of diabetic men who have had the disease for many years, who suffer from neuropathy, and probably have not maintained very good control, are plagued with sexual dysfunction. Above the age of fifty-five, the likelihood of having difficulties with erection occurs in about 70 percent of men with diabetes, and at seventy, about 95 percent.

Though sexual difficulties can obviously be psychological (and often the anxiety about the possibility of future problems can cause them), in most cases an organic dysfunction quite specific to diabetes is the reason for an increased incidence of impotence at an earlier age than the rest of the population.

What occurs is not loss of libido or desire for sexual gratification, but the ability to have an erection. This ability may gradually diminish and eventually vanish completely. Usually the cause is damage to the nerves and blood vessels that control an erection. This is almost always associated with other neuropathies, often in the legs and feet and, most likely, the bladder.

Occasionally the reason is an obstruction or clot in one of the blood vessels supplying the penis, and some-

times poorly controlled diabetes causes temporary impotence as a result of a general weakened condition.

IS IMPOTENCE IN THE CARDS?

Though some studies have been made, it is still uncertain just how many diabetic men eventually develop
sexual problems by middle age. Uncertain, too, is whether
impotence is related to the severity of the diabetes. Undoubtedly it is affected by the quality of blood-sugar
control over the years, and the number of years since the
diagnosis was made.

This does not mean that impotence is in the cards for
every male diabetic—there are men who have had diabetes for fifty years and have no problem—nor that all is
lost and nothing can be done about it.

First, it must be determined whether your impotence,
which never happens suddenly but comes about gradually when it is caused by diabetes, is psychological or
physiological. Your internist will suggest an examination by a urologist and perhaps a neurologist, and if
there is no obvious physical reason for the problem, may
suggest an NPT (nocturnal penile tumescence) assessment. This is usually performed in the sleep-disorder department of a large medical center, and monitors the
nocturnal erections that normally occur at regular intervals while a man sleeps. If you have normal nocturnal
erections, then you are not suffering from nerve or vascular damage, and psychological counseling will probably be recommended. If your neuropathy is the culprit,
you will not have erections in your sleep or at any other
time.

Obviously, if your impotence is the result of poor diabetic control, then good control is your answer.

If the cause is vascular obstruction, sometimes surgery can make a dramatic difference.

DEALING WITH THE PROBLEM

When impotence is caused by neuropathy, there is a choice of treatments available today and one of them may work for you. First, ask your doctor to check your testosterone level to see if you are producing a normal amount. If not, you can take supplemental testosterone by mouth, injection, or skin patch (Androderm) and see if it enhances your libido and the ability to maintain an erection.

Other remedies include drugs, implants, injections, pumps, and more. A urologist who specializes in problems of impotency can explain the merits of each and the possibilities that one of them will be helpful for you.

Penis-enlarging drugs, Viagra, Cialis, and Levitra, have proved to be a boon to many men, diabetics and otherwise. If you fail on one of them, try another and it may produce the desired result. They are taken by pill about an hour before needed and enhance the response to sexual stimulation.

When these drugs are ineffective or deemed unsuitable for you, there are other nonsurgical treatments to try, such as injections into the penis of a drug called Caverject that contains prostaglandins.

And finally, yohimbine, available as an herb or a prescription drug, has been found to be helpful for some men.

Though there is no way to repair damaged nerve endings, you may want to look into the possibility of a penile implant or an inflatable device, both of which are designed to allow sexual intercourse complete with ejaculation and orgasm. When you have an implant, flexible silicone rods are placed in the penis, making it rigid enough for intercourse. A problem is that the penis remains rigid.

The more complex "inflatable erectile prosthesis" allows actual simulation of a natural erection by the implantation of a device that inflates and deflates the penis on demand by squeezing a pump.

Another possible helpful aid is a vacuum constriction device that gives the penis rigidity. This is a noninvasive technique and may be worth a try before resorting to implants.

EFFECTS ON FERTILITY

Diabetes doesn't affect a man's ability to produce sperm, so, assuming he is not impotent, there's usually no reason he cannot father children. Sometimes, though, diabetic neuropathy will cause a condition known as "retrograde ejaculation." Because the nerve supply to the penis is impaired, the sphincters won't open and the semen, including the sperm, drops back into the bladder. This doesn't interfere with intercourse or orgasm, but obviously precludes fertility.

SEX AND THE DIABETIC WOMAN

Diabetic women tend to have more sexual difficulties than women with normal blood sugar, often experiencing a marked reduction in lubrication and sometimes in their sexual desire and ability to have orgasms. This is especially true when they have peripheral nerve damage that diminishes sensation. If you are experiencing such problems, try taking vitamin B complex every day and ask your doctor about the new drugs now available for treating neuropathy (see Chapter 10).

Women with diabetes may also have other related problems as a result of lowered glucose tolerance.

One is an increased tendency toward vaginal and urinary infections. When your glucose levels are high, your vagina provides the perfect environment for problems. Yeast especially loves the glucose found in vaginal secretions and many a case of diabetes has been first detected in the gynecologist's office. Add to that the sometimes diminished ability of the white cells to rally around and fight infections. If you notice any signs of vaginal or urinary infection, get yourself to your doctor immediately. There are drugs that can alleviate them, usually in short order. Along with the drugs, however, you must get your diabetes back in good control and keep it there.

Vaginal dryness is another problem that often accompanies poorly controlled diabetes. This will improve along with better control and, in the meantime, can be counteracted by the use of a personal lubricant made for this purpose, such as K-Y Jelly, Astroglide, or Surgilube. By the way, never use a lubricant that is not designed for vaginal use. Most cosmetic creams, for example, contain ingredients that can irritate tender tissues. Don't use petroleum jelly or oil because it may cake and dry, provide a habitat for bacteria, and block the release of your own secretions as well. The only exception is vitamin E oil, which doesn't dry and may possibly have a beneficial effect on the vaginal lining.

Even more effective than lubricants are nonhormonal vaginal moisturizing gels, including Replens and Gyne-Moistrin, now sold over the counter. They help by plumping up the cells of the vaginal lining with moisture, making it less dry and irritable. They should not be used as lubricants, however, but inserted into the vagina about three times a week, preferably in the morning. If you need a lubricant, too, use it just before intercourse.

WHAT KIND OF CONTRACEPTION?

For the diabetic, probably the best contraceptive methods are the mechanical kinds—the diaphragm or the condom. These usually present no problems, as long as you remember to use them every time, unless you are prone to fungal infections. If you do get these infections frequently, try using a condom with a spermicidal foam that has an acidic component to discourage fungus.

Birth-control pills are not the best idea for several reasons. Most important, some studies have shown that the hormones in the pill can lower your glucose tolerance and raise your insulin needs. If you do use them, choose combination estrogen-progesterone pills with the lowest dose and potency of progestin available. Keep a close watch on your glucose to be sure it is not affected and stay in touch with your doctors.

Many physicians think that the IUD, the intrauterine device, is associated with increased vaginal infections. Diabetics need no more ways of acquiring infections. In addition, according to researchers, there is a high failure (pregnancy) rate among diabetic IUD users, probably because of an unusual metabolic interaction of the device with the endometrium, the uterine lining.

For those couples who do not want children or have completed their families, sterilization is an option.

CHANGES IN INSULIN NEEDS

For many women, insulin requirements change the week before their menstrual period, so you should check your blood and respond accordingly. Your pattern of needing more or less insulin at that time will usually remain consistent.

IF YOU USE AN INSULIN PUMP

Obviously, it can be uncomfortable to have sexual intercourse while wearing an insulin pump. If you can't find a satisfactory position, it won't hurt you to detach it for a while, just as you do when you take a bath.

SEX AFTER MENOPAUSE

Because menopause decreases the estrogen circulating throughout your body, uncomfortable vaginal changes may become even more bothersome, especially for diabetics and more so for those with premature menopause. Type 1 diabetics often have early menopause, sometimes even before the age of forty, giving them more time to develop problems.

After menopause, natural lubrication decreases, along with sensory perception. The vagina becomes dryer, narrower, and less pliable and expandable. Its lining loses its tough protective layer of cornified cells and becomes thinner, smoother, less elastic, less acidic, and more easily irritated and susceptible to infections. An easily irritated and inflamed lining can obviously lead to a minimal interest in sex.

If you don't want these changes to affect your attitude

toward making love, you are going to have to deal with them one way or another. Don't be afraid to discuss your problems with your gynecologist. Be open and frank so you can get on with your sex life.

Try the lubricants and moisturizers and, if they don't help enough, consider hormone replacement therapy. Your best bet is vaginal estrogen cream that is applied topically and is considered quite safe as a short-term therapy. It may be used briefly and temporarily to relieve the worst symptoms and infections that refuse to respond to anything else. When the tissues are restored, then you should use it only as needed. Very little estrogen is absorbed into the bloodstream when you use the cream but, on the other hand, it is still hormone therapy, so you must report to your gynecologist regularly.

15

TRAVELING: DIABETICS ON THE MOVE

If you are just a beginner at this business of being a diabetic, you probably are afraid to travel. You feel much safer at home. You are not interested in surprises, not when you're away from your own kitchen, your own medicine cabinet, and especially your own doctor.

But once you have learned the rules, whether it involves only diet or includes insulin or pills, and you have had sufficient practice coping with the variations of a diabetic life, then there is no reason you cannot travel anywhere in this world like anyone else. But you must remember, just because you're breathing the pure mountain air of the Alps or savoring the sights of Hong Kong, you have not left your diabetes behind you. It travels with you. So the same rules apply wherever you are.

There are a few precautions that a person with diabetes, especially one who is insulin-dependent, should take. Let's run through them briefly. If you are not yet an experienced traveler, you may want to slip this book into your luggage for handy reference.

A BEFORE-YOU-GO LIST OF SUGGESTIONS

• Don't travel (and that means anywhere, including the next town) without some visible medical identification affixed to your person. Wear a bracelet or necklace stating "I am a diabetic," and carry two cards (one in your pocket, another in your wallet) that say the same and also list your medication and allergies, along with your name, address, and phone number. If possible, carry a card in the language of the country you are visiting.

• Before leaving town, go to your doctor for a checkup to be sure you are in good shape for your venture. Don't go anywhere when your condition isn't stable. Get checked out by your dentist, too, so that you don't find yourself in Tanzania with a toothache and a blood-sugar level that's askew. Go to your podiatrist, because you will undoubtedly be doing a lot of walking and you should be sure there is no foot trouble brewing.

• Take along an extra pair of eyeglasses, or at least a copy of your prescription. Many a person, not necessarily diabetic, has toured Europe out of focus after losing his/her only pair of glasses the first week out.

• Have any necessary inoculations long before your departure date, so any reactions to them will be over before your trip. Sometimes the shots affect your diabetic equilibrium.

• Take enough of all your medications to get you through your entire trip, along with an extra supply just in case your return home is delayed. Keep them in their original containers with the proper labels and take copies of your prescriptions that note the brand and generic names of each drug. Pack them in your carry-on bag, along with your doctor's contact information and extra prescriptions. Be prepared in case you have to stay on the road longer than you anticipated.

BE PREPARED FOR PROBLEMS

• Ask your doctor to prescribe an antidiarrheal medication to take along, just in case you'll need it. Lomotil and Imodium are effective for treating the symptoms. Antibiotics such as Bactrim or Cipro will help prevent or treat the disease itself.

If you are going to a country where you are fairly sure to run into intestinal problems, pack some Pepto-Bismol tablets and take one tablet four times a day as a preventive. Don't be frightened if your tongue and stool turn black.

Also take along an antiemetic to prevent or treat nausea. If you are susceptible to motion sickness, take the preventive four hours *before* you board the boat, walk into the airplane, or step into the car. Be sure to take along some antiemetic medication in suppository form in case you can't keep anything down. Remember, too, that medicine like Compazine, effective against nausea, can be injected with your insulin syringe.

• Carry in your pocket or handbag a signed note from your physician stating that you are a diabetic and require insulin and syringes. That's so the customs inspectors, coming upon a supply of syringes, won't suspect they have discovered a drug addict who must be turned over to the gendarmes. The statement will also help you buy more syringes if you need them. Make sure the note explains your current treatment and lists any other medications you take in addition to insulin.

• Take more than enough oral agents or insulin and syringes *for the entire trip*. Always include a bottle of fast-acting insulin, even if you normally take only Intermediate insulin or none at all. In an emergency, this will be essential.

• A pen injector or a syringe prefilled with insulin may be more convenient when you're on the move.

• Take plenty of blood-glucose testing equipment. Take a glucose meter and use it to test your blood as usual. Meters are small and light today.

• If you use an insulin pump, include extra pump supplies and don't forget the user manual. Talk to your doctor about resetting the pump if you are changing time zones. Just in case, take insulin and syringes, too.

• Try a hospital emergency room if you have problems getting supplies away from home.

DON'T BE CAUGHT SHORT

• Unopened insulin need not be refrigerated. It will survive nicely for a few months in any environment that's comfortable for you. Do not use insulin that has been exposed to very hot temperatures (don't let it sit in the sun or in a closed car) or has been frozen. This means it must *not* be packed in your luggage if you fly, because temperatures are often below freezing in the baggage compartments. Oral hypoglycemic agents are not harmed by freezing, however.

• Carry your oral agents or insulin and syringes *with you* in your hand luggage to cover those possible occasions when you go one way and your luggage goes another. This is important. It won't be harmed by the airport X-ray machines. Disposable insulin syringes may be used more than once. Seven syringes can be adequate for two weeks. After use, simply recap the needle. Also carry *with you* your insulin pump infusion sets, lancets, glucose meter, glucagon kit, glucose gel or tablets, blood and ketone test strips. And don't forget some snacks.

• If you take insulin, carrying your own is especially

important. In many countries, only U-40 is available. But don't panic if you run short—it's really quite simple to convert your usual dose to U-40 (see Chapter 6).

• Your brand of insulin will probably be available in other countries, but carry more than enough of your own, just in case you can't find it.

• A good thing to remember is that 1-cc tuberculin syringes can be substituted for U-100 syringes where each line equals one unit of insulin.

• If you take oral agents and need to buy more, you will find counterparts available in foreign countries.

SPEAKING THEIR LANGUAGE

• If you are going somewhere where a language other than your own is spoken, memorize in the appropriate language (and write in clear lettering on a card) the following phrases: "I am a diabetic." "Sugar or orange juice, please." "Please get me a doctor."

Here they are in four languages:

I am a diabetic.
French: *Je suis diabétique.*
Spanish: *Yo soy diabético.*
German: *Ich bin zuckerkrank.*
Italian: *Io sono diabètico.*

Sugar or orange juice, please.
French: *Sucre ou jus d'orange, s'il vous plaît.*
Spanish: *Azúcar o un vaso de jugo de naranja, por favor.*
German: *Zucker oder Orangensaft, bitte.*
Italian: *Zucchero o succo di arància, per favore.*

Please get me a doctor.
French: *Allez chercher un médecin, si'il vous plaît.*
Spanish: *Haga me el favor de llamar al médico.*
German: *Rufen Sie bitte einen Arzt.*
Italian: *Per favore chiami un dottore.*

• Another precaution before you leave home: Though you certainly hope it won't happen in the middle of a great vacation, there's always the possibility of getting sick and needing a doctor, whether you are diabetic or not. It is always best to be prepared. Write to the American Diabetes Association (1701 N. Beauregard St., Alexandria, VA 22311), call 800-342-2383, or go to www.diabetes.org for a list of affiliate or chapter offices of the Association wherever you plan to travel within the United States. If you need a doctor in Cleveland, for example, a call to the Cleveland Diabetes Association will get you a list of local doctors experienced in diabetic care.

From the same national ADA office or from the British Diabetic Association (10 Queen Anne Street, London W1M OBD, England), you can get a list of diabetes associations in foreign countries. (Telephone: London 011-44-171-637-3644.)

When you arrive at your destination, remember that the U.S. embassy or consulate will supply the names of English-speaking physicians upon request. So will the major hotels.

Another suggestion: Well before you leave on a trip to a foreign country, send for a list of English-speaking physicians all over the world, and information on climate, food, and sanitary conditions from the free, nonprofit International Association for Medical Assistance to Travellers (IAMAT, 417 Center Street, Lewiston, NY 14092. 716-754-4883; www.IAMAT.org).

TRAVEL TIPS ON YOUR WAY

Now you have finally had all the proper checkups, your diabetes is under excellent control, you have gathered your supplies together, tucked away all those lists and statements. You are ready to get your show on the road. *And* you do not want to hear any more advice. However, we have a few more tips, all designed to make it easier for the traveler who happens to have diabetes.

CHANGING TIME ZONES

Most people who take medication for diabetes are concerned about their schedules for insulin or pills when they cross time zones (traveling north or south requires no adjustments). When you travel by car or ship, no problem. The time changes are so gradual they will not affect your timetable. Simply take your medication at your usual hour according to the time it is wherever you are.

If you take oral agents, do the same, even if you fly long distances, crossing many time zones. Take the pills according to your new time.

But when you fly long distances into new time zones and you take insulin, it gets a little trickier. Here's how to handle it.

Keep your watch set at your point-of-departure time, so you will know how many hours have passed since your last injection. Eat your meals and snacks on your normal schedule, according to the time on your watch. If you have requested special meals or mealtimes when you made your reservations, confirm this 24 hours before the flight, and remind the flight attendant when you board the plane that you must have your meals on time because you are a diabetic. If meals at different times from those of the other passengers seem to be too difficult to arrange, board the plane with your own box of food. (And, of course, you have not set forth without your usual emergency snack supplies.)

On arrival, if *more* than 24 hours have passed since your last injection, take a few *extra* units of fast-acting insulin and/or Intermediate insulin. However, if *less* than 24 hours have passed since your last injection, take *fewer* units of Intermediate-acting insulin because some of the dose you took the previous day is still in your bloodstream. If you are skipping a meal, you must adjust for less food.

After taking your insulin, set your watch to the time of the place in which you now find yourself, and start taking your injections accordingly.

GOING FROM WEST TO EAST

When you are traveling east, perhaps from the United States to Europe, your day will be *less* than 24 hours long and you will require less insulin. Suppose you have your insulin shot at 7 A.M. on the day of departure. You leave New York at 6 P.M. and arrive in Europe at 2 A.M. our time. But it is 8 A.M. European time. Breakfast will have been served on the plane before landing. Do not eat it. And do not take your morning insulin at that time. Instead, take it at noon just before lunch when it is about 24 hours from the time you took your last shot.

Do not take your second shot before dinner because your day has been condensed and you don't want to overdose—you could end up in the hospital with an insulin reaction instead of on a tour bus having a fine time.

Now set your watch to European time. The next morning, take your usual dose.

Remember to adjust your insulin to your physical activity. If you will be much more active than you normally are at home, you must compensate by taking a few less units of insulin or eating more food (see Chapter 6).

GOING FROM EAST TO WEST

Now, what about going the other way, from east to west when your first day of travel will be *more* than 24 hours? Let's use this example: You take your insulin and depart from Europe at 8 A.M. You arrive in New York seven hours later at 3 P.M. European time, 10 A.M. New York time.

Keep your watch set on foreign time. You have had breakfast before getting on the plane, and you have eaten lunch during the flight. Your next meal is dinner at 6 P.M. European time but noon in New York. Eat your dinner then. Eat your bedtime snack at 11 P.M. European time, 7 P.M. in New York.

Go to bed early. When you wake up, you are five hours late for your next shot. Take a little more of your fast-acting insulin and your usual dose of NPH, Lantus, or Levemir. If you are not on fast insulin, take your usual dose of NPH, Lantus, or Levemir and eat less starch for breakfast.

• Never make a move without your cache of emergency carbohydrates. You must have this *with* you at all times, just on the chance—however remote it may be in your case—that you will have a hypoglycemic reaction. Sugar cubes, candies, cookies, crackers. Don't carry sugar-free candies; they won't help you a bit if you have low blood sugar.

• If you are traveling by car, and especially if you are the driver, take the equivalent of 10 grams of carbohydrate every hour: two graham crackers, an orange, 15 grapes, whatever.

NOW YOU ARE THERE

Once you have arrived at your destination, simply start living in your accustomed way, adjusting your medication to your blood-sugar level and your physical activity just as you would at home.

A few things to keep in mind:

• You may be much more active on vacation than you are in everyday life. If you are going to do strenuous sightseeing, play tennis, ski, swim, anything that burns up considerable sugar, you will require more food or less insulin. Oral agents are not so critical and do not have to be adjusted. On the other hand, if you overindulge, you cannot expect an extra pill to correct it, as you would if you were on insulin and took an extra dose when your sugar was high.

Suppose you are an insulin user and you plan to play a few tough sets of singles, make a cross-country ski trek, or even do some heavy sightseeing on foot.

Check your blood. If it is low, eat extra carbohydrate and protein before setting off. If it is high, have some carbohydrate after about an hour of exercise. Or reduce your insulin as an added precaution against reactions. Sometimes you will need snacks every half hour or so of heavy exercise. Try to avoid strenuous exercise when your insulin is peaking (see Chapter 6).

• Never ski, swim, bike, hike, or climb alone, but always rely on the buddy system. If you should have a reaction, your buddy will cope with it if you have explained what to do. Unless you started off with high sugar, the exertion may drop your blood sugar very quickly to subnormal levels.

• At high altitudes, the symptoms of altitude mountain sickness (AMS) can mimic those of hypoglycemic reactions, perhaps making you feel lightheaded, weak, confused, shaky, breathless. Are you suffering from AMS or low sugar? You will know only by testing your sugar at that very moment. Don't wait.

• Be prepared for delays when you travel. You never know when a traffic jam, a delayed flight, or a missed connection will mess up your schedule. Carry some snacks and drinks with you. Be prepared to make adjustments in your medication and meals.

KEEP YOUR SHOES ON!

• If you have foot problems, *never* go barefoot, even on the beach. One sharp shell can get you into long-term trouble. Don't get sunburned. A burn is a burn, and the stress it causes can throw off your control.

Use foot powder, wash your feet, and change your socks frequently. Keep an eye on your feet, giving them a daily inspection. Unaccustomed walking can produce blisters and rubs, especially if you are wearing new shoes, which you should *not* be doing. Do not let any foot injuries get even the slightest bit out of control. Rest your feet, take the pressure off, wear sneakers, sandals, or slippers if necessary, and if trouble seems to be brewing, see a doctor *immediately,* not two weeks after you have returned home.

• Watch what you eat. Nobody wants a gastrointestinal upset, but diabetics can have their whole vacation ruined by the after-effects and the difficulty of getting their blood sugar back under control. In tropical countries, don't eat raw vegetables, soft cheese, ice cream, rare meats, cream sauces, fruits you can't peel. Use bottled or boiled water even for brushing your teeth. Don't drink fresh milk or water, and avoid ice cubes. One man bought an unpeeled melon in India, thinking he could eat it safely once it was skinned. But his host served it to him cut up and floating in ice water. He had his melon, plus a good case of amebiasis and diarrhea.

• If you get up late and miss breakfast, take about 20 percent less insulin because you'll be having only two meals that day. Don't try to make up for the lost meal by eating more now, because that will present you with too much carbohydrate to handle at one time.

DEALING WITH NEW CUSTOMS

• In some countries—Spain, for example—the dinner hour is late. If you plan to have your meal at the fashionable hour of, say, 10 P.M., then you must prepare in advance. There are two ways to handle this situation. Either take less insulin in the morning and give yourself a second shot before going to bed. Or consume the major portion of your carbohydrate allowance (the equivalent of two slices of bread) at 6 P.M., then eat everything else—your main course, vegetables, dessert—at dinner. Of course, you will then skip the carbohydrates at the table—rice, corn, potatoes, bread, etc. And don't eat your bedtime snack either. This also applies to weddings and other parties here at home.

• Be sure your traveling companions know how to cope with both hypoglycemia (low sugar) and hyperglycemia (high sugar). Your companions should know that you need quick sugar if you are having an insulin reaction—granulated sugar, honey, a soft drink (not a diet drink), candy, orange juice, etc., followed shortly thereafter by some protein. Or you may be given "instant glucose" or cake icing, which comes in toothpaste-like tubes and can be forced through the lips. If this isn't quickly effective, a subcutaneous shot of glucagon and a doctor may be necessary. Have all the supplies always handy (see Chapter 8).

If you are suffering from *high* sugar *and* acetone, then you need insulin and perhaps the service of a doctor.

• Adjust the eating customs of the places you visit to your own needs. This means making sure you get the right proportions of carbohydrate, protein, and fat, no matter where you are. A continental breakfast, for example—a roll and coffee—isn't going to be enough for you unless that is what you normally consume at home. Order additional food. Many foods, notably a lot of Chinese and Japanese dishes, contain sugar and must be avoided. Sukiyaki, for example, is made with sugar or sweet wine.

Remember your carbohydrate exchanges: 1 cup of rice is the equivalent of 2 slices of bread, or 30 grams of carbohydrate. So is one regular-size pita, even if it is as flat as a pancake. Some tropical fruits, such as mangos, are very high in sugar. Check them out before eating them freely.

• Test your blood glucose after you've eaten a food that you're not accustomed to eating. If the effect is to raise your sugar inordinately, avoid that food in the future.

• Wines and liquors needn't be avoided, if you drink them in moderation, as you do at home (see pages 91–94).

• If you happen to get sick away from home, treat

yourself just as you would in your natural habitat (see Chapter 11). Test your blood four times a day for sugar and if it's high, check your urine for acetone. *Always take your insulin.* If your sugar is low *and* you can't eat, take half your usual dose of insulin. If your sugar is high, whether you can eat or not, take your regular amount. Always take your normal dosage of oral agents unless your sugar is very low, under 100 mgs.

If you have high sugar and are vomiting, take your full insulin dose. Then take an antiemetic by suppository. Eat or drink some carbohydrate every hour—perhaps 3 ounces of orange juice mixed with water, or 3 ounces of ginger ale (*not* sugar-free), or ice cream, toast, broth, cereal, etc. Don't tough it out—if you need a doctor, get one.

TRAVELING IS FUN, REMEMBER?

With all these precautions and pieces of advice, perhaps you think it might be simpler to stay home. But make all your preparations, keep the advice in the back of your mind just in case you need it, and go forth, not to worry, but to enjoy yourself. You take your diabetes with you, but other people take their problems with them, too, and may not be as carefree as they seem. Enjoy.

16

CAN DIABETES BE PREVENTED?

STOPPING DIABETES IN ITS TRACKS

You are not destined to be a type 2 diabetic, even if the disease runs in your family—nor are your relatives. This is a disease that can almost always be delayed, prevented, or even reversed, usually with simple lifestyle changes and sometimes the help of drugs.

The more scientists have learned about diabetes, the more they have been focusing on its very earliest stages—insulin resistance, the metabolic syndrome, and prediabetes—and searching for ways to nip it in the bud before it becomes a big problem down the road.

Perhaps it is too late for you, but here is information and advice for family and friends who are not diabetics but are are at risk.

ARE YOU INSULIN RESISTANT?

If your body doesn't respond effectively enough to insulin—even if you make plenty of it yourself—you are insulin resistant. Insulin facilitates the delivery of glucose to the cells, where it provides the fuel for energy. When that process is not in good working order, the excess glucose can't get into your body's cells and instead builds up in your bloodstream, giving you an elevated blood-sugar level.

DO YOU HAVE METABOLIC SYNDROME?

The metabolic syndrome is a cluster of risk factors that sow the seeds for diabetes. They include an elevated fasting glucose level, high blood pressure, high triglycerides, low HDL cholesterol, and obesity (especially around the middle). A third to a half of those who have this combination of risk factors eventually develop diabetes.

Because of the metabolic syndrome, more children than ever before are becoming diabetic, and experts are warning that many others are headed down the same path. A recent study from the University of Kansas showed that out of 375 second- and third-grade students, 5 percent had metabolic syndrome and 45 percent had one or two of its risk factors.

ARE YOU PREDIABETIC?

When your blood-glucose levels are higher than normal, yet not high enough to qualify you as a bona fide diabetic, you have prediabetes (formerly known as impaired glucose tolerance)—and the earlier you get on its case, the better. If you don't do something about it *now,* you're looking for trouble later. More and more specialists today agree that prediabetics must be identified much earlier than ever thought before and that *treatment must start immediately.*

If your fasting glucose level measures anywhere between 100 and 125 mg/dl (above that, you are diabetic), or your A1c values are 5.3 percent or above, you have prediabetes, or impaired glucose tolerance. That means that your blood-sugar control system is out of whack and, along with about 41 million other Americans age forty to seventy-four, you have a 30 percent chance of developing type 2 diabetes within 3 years, and a 50 percent or greater chance within 10 years. Meanwhile, some long-term damage to the body may have already been done. For example, the U.S. Department of Health and Human Services warns that prediabetes increases the risk of heart disease by 50 percent.

By the way, you probably won't suspect you have a problem because, other than a large waistline, symptoms are rare. So it is an excellent idea to have your doctor test for it every year, especially if you are overweight, over the age of forty-five, and have diabetic relatives.

CHANGING THE ODDS

You can stop or slow down the diabetic clock by getting on your own case. Remember that the very same lifestyle changes that help diabetics fight their high blood sugar are the best way to treat prediabetes. A recent study found that weight loss, diet, and exercise cut the incidence of diabetes among prediabetics almost twice as effectively as medication.

First, you can lose some weight if you are too heavy. You can get into a regular exercise routine. You can switch to a low-fat diet, avoid fast-food restaurants, and cut down on refined carbohydrates, such as white bread, white rice, soft drinks and sodas, starchy vegetables, and sweets.

Second, if necessary, you can use other weapons, too, perhaps an insulin-sensitizing medication such as metformin (Glucophage), one of the TZDs, or Acarbose. Changes in lifestyle *plus* the right medication can improve your odds even more dramatically.

Here's a list of ways to hold back the onset of diabetes or even prevent type 2 diabetes altogether. Some have been proven to work, others are thought to work. None of them will hurt you, so it's worth giving them a try.

DROP A FEW POUNDS

The most important change you can make if you are too heavy is to lose weight, especially if you carry much of your extra fat around your waistline. Nine out of ten newly diagnosed diabetics are overweight, according to the CDC. The results of a six-year Diabetes Prevention Program on 3,000 prediabetics (59 percent obese; 30 percent overweight) revealed that even a small weight loss—5 to 7 percent—deters diabetes by 58 percent.

The prevalence of overweight youngsters has doubled in the past two decades, accompanied by an epidemic of type 2 diabetes diagnosed in childhood.

The fat that accumulates around the waist and abdomen is a good indicator of the risk for getting type 2, for both children and adults. According to a study of 27,000 men conducted over thirteen years and reported in 2005, men whose waists are 37.9 to 39.8 inches have a risk five times as great as those whose waists are 34 inches or less. Those whose waists are 40 to 62 inches have twelve times the risk.

GET MOVING

It's not necessary to become a marathon runner to lower your chances of diabetes, but if you get up off the couch and start exercising, you will improve your body's ability to metabolize sugar. Try to get into the habit of doing some variety of moderate aerobic exercise for a minimum of 30 minutes a day at least three, preferably five, times a week. Exercise not only burns up blood sugar but it also helps you lose weight and stay fit.

Researchers have analyzed data from the well-known nurses' health study, which surveyed over 70,000 nurses age forty to sixty-five who did not have diabetes in 1986. During eight years of follow-up, they confirmed 1,419 cases of type 2. After adjusting for many factors, they concluded that the women who were consistently active during the eight years had 41 percent less risk for diabetes than the women who were consistently sedentary.

When it comes to exercise, more is better, and even walking just a few times a week is a lot better than nothing.

IMPROVE YOUR DIET

If you have a genetic suceptibility to diabetes and above-normal blood sugar, even though it's not high enough to make you a diabetic, avoid sugar and simple carbohydrates such as sweets, regular soft drinks and sodas, huge plates of pasta, and certain kinds of fruit. Instead, stoke up on complex carbohydrates, which include grains, starches, some vegetables, and legumes. See pages 42 to 47 to see what they are.

Sugar-sweetened soft drinks and fruit punches provide excessive calories and rapidly absorbable sugar that can result in weight gain and diabetes. Soft drinks are the leading source of added sugars in the U.S. diet, according to a study published in the *Journal of the American Medical Association* in 2004, because they contain large amounts of high-fructose corn syrup—the equivalent of 18 teaspoons of refined sugar per bottle or can.

Fast food, too, is notorious for causing many Americans to be overweight. A survey has shown that people who go to fast-food restaurants at least twice a week have about twice the incidence of metabolic syndrome and prediabetes as those who don't.

CUT BACK ON RED MEAT AND HOT DOGS

The connection between a diet high in red meat and processed meats and type 2 diabetes was made way back in 1952 in my own study in medical school, when we found that rats fed high-fat diets developed much higher glucose levels than other rats. Fifty years later, current studies show that people who eat a lot of fatty red meat are those with the highest incidence of diabetes.

Hot dogs, bacon, lunch meats, and fatty fast foods are the worst, according to an investigation reported in 2004 by researchers at Harvard Medical School. The study followed over 37,000 women age forty-five or older for an average of eight years and found that women who ate five or more servings of red meat a week had a 29 percent increase in diabetes risk compared with women who ate red meat less than once a week. Five or more servings of processed meats a week raised the risk to 43 percent.

Iron may play a role also. Red and processed meats are high in iron, and some research has shown that people who get the most iron in their diets were much more likely to develop diabetes.

ADD THESE FOODS AND SUPPLEMENTS

Certain foods may help control blood sugar. Among them are:

• **Coffee.** Several studies show that heavy coffee drinkers are less likely to develop diabetes. Research in the Netherlands showed a drop in risk of diabetes by more than 50 percent for men and 30 percent for women who drank four or five cups a day. Then, in

2006, a study at the University of Minnesota of almost 29,000 postmenopausal women showed that those who drank six or more cups of regular or decaffeinated coffee a day had a 33 percent reduced risk of type 2 diabetes, compared with those who drank none. Surprisingly, the link with a reduced risk was even stronger for decaffeinated coffee, so the effect may be attributed to a variety of minerals, antioxidants, and phytochemical compounds that may slow down the release of glucose from the liver.

That doesn't mean you should start drinking a pot of java a day, however. Wait until more results come in.

• **Alcohol.** Having a drink or two a day may reduce the risk of getting type 2 diabetes, concluded several recent studies. Moderate drinking is also associated with a lowered risk of heart disease. One theory is that the polyphenols in alcohol decrease insulin resistance. By the way, it doesn't matter whether you're imbibing hard liquor, wine, or beer. It all counts.

• **Dark chocolate** may lower your blood pressure and improve insulin resistance because it contains flavonoids, say researchers at Tufts University in Boston. On the other hand, keep in mind that you're adding calories.

• **Spices,** such as black pepper, cloves, bay leaves, and especially cinnamon, contain substances that help with blood-sugar control. A small study in Pakistan found that cinnamon seemed to reduce fasting glucose levels by as much as 29 percent, and German researchers came up with data that supported this claim, showing that about a teaspoon of cinnamon per day had a positive effect on blood sugar. And scientists at the USDA's Beltsville Human Nutrition Research Center found a natural compound in cinnamon that they think may have insulin-like properties.

• **Magnesium.** Magnesium-rich foods like spinach and other leafy-green vegetables, whole grains, seafood, and nuts may reduce your diabetes risk. That said, magnesium supplements can be harmful if you have kidney disease.

• **High-fiber foods.** Research from the University of Toronto reported in 2004 that eating a high-fiber cereal may help prevent type 2 diabetes by lowering insulin resistance. And a team of doctors at the University of Minnesota who followed nearly 36,000 older women for six years found that those who ate more whole-grain foods and dietary fiber had a lower risk of diabetes.

GET MORE SLEEP

Late to bed and early to rise gives you circles under your eyes and also increases your risk of converting from prediabetes to diabetes. The findings of a group of physicians at Boston University associated short sleep with impaired glucose tolerance and heart attacks. They suggest getting seven or eight hours of sleep a night.

TAKE FISH OIL

A compound found in fish oil may help stave off diabetes by improving the body's response to insulin. It has long been known that populations that eat a lot of fish containing omega-3 fatty acids, such as tuna, salmon, and mackerel, have lower rates of type 2 diabetes than those who eat less. That fact led to a trial of daily supplements of an omega-3 fatty acid on a small group of insulin-resistant people who ended up with a significant decrease in insulin resistance. There are plenty of fish-oil supplements on the market but none has been scientifically tested, so it is not known if they are safe. A new drug called Omacor is a high-powered form of omega-3 fatty acids. Be sure to consult your doctor before taking any fish-oil supplements because they are anticoagulants and may thin your blood too much.

TEST FOR NAFD

Many physicians are unaware of a syndrome that affects people, prediabetics among them, who, left untreated, will ultimately develop diabetes or severe liver disease. The syndrome is Nonalcoholic Fatty-liver Disease (NAFD), a condition that can lead to diabetes and cirrhosis. The syndrome is detected via abdominal ultrasound that reveals the liver is filled with fat. NAFD can lead to Nonalcoholic Stentohepatitis (NASH), which is inflammation and fibrosis of the liver.

DRUGS THAT FIGHT PREDIABETES

METFORMIN

The best news in recent history for high-risk prediabetics are the insulin-sensitizing drugs called metformin (sold under the brand name Glucophage) and the oral agents Avandia and Actos, both TZDs. Metformin suppresses the liver's production of glucose that would otherwise pour into your bloodstream. In addition, it lowers levels of LDL cholesterol and triglycerides. And, miracle of miracles, it does not promote weight gain. It is taken for life, unless you lose weight and have a significant decrease in insulin resistance.

Usually taken once or twice a day with food, metformin has become—along with lifestyle changes—the primary weapon in the war against diabetes. The Diabetes Prevention Program study found that people who take metformin can reduce their risk by 31 percent.

TZDS

Right now, researchers are studying the likely possibility that TZDs, the oral agents called Avandia and Actos, can perform the same miracle of preventing or delaying diabetes.

ACARBOSE (PRECOSE)

This is another drug that can be used to reduce the number of prediabetics who go on to become diabetics. In 2002, an international trial reported that a group of patients whose glucose levels were above normal, but not sufficiently elevated to be diagnosed as diabetics, could reduce their risk by taking Precose as a preventive.

OTHER HELPFUL DRUGS

• Cholesterol-fighting medications such as the statins and the fibrates will reduce your LDL and triglyceride levels, providing another way to lower your blood sugar and your risk.

• A blood-pressure drug, ramipril (Altace), has been found to reduce the chance of developing diabetes.

• Aspirin and aspirin-like drugs may keep diabetes in check because they reduce low-level inflammation that disrupts the body's ability to process insulin, possibly triggering type 2.

CAUTION: Do not take any of the above medications, including aspirin, without consulting your doctor.

RESOURCES

For additional information and help, here is a list of resources that will answer questions, send general information and literature, and provide referrals as well as the addresses, telephone numbers, and websites of their local affiliates or chapters.

American Diabetes Association, 1701 N. Beauregard Street, Alexandria, VA 22311; 800-342-2383; www.diabetes.org.

International Diabetes Federation (IDF), Avenue Emile de Mot 19, 1000 Brussels, Belgium; www.idf.org.

Joslin Diabetes Center, 1 Joslin Place, Boston, MA 02215; 617-732-2400; www.joslin.org.

Juvenile Diabetes Research Foundation International, 120 Wall Street, New York, NY 10005; 800-533-2873; www.jdrf.org.

National Diabetes Education Program, 1 Diabetes Way, Bethesda, MD 20814; 800-438-5383; www.ndep.nih.gov.

INDEX

ABOUT THE AUTHORS

STANLEY MIRSKY, M.D., F.A.C.P., Diplomate of Internal Medicine, is associate clinical professor of metabolic diseases at the Mount Sinai School of Medicine in New York, and is on the staffs of Mount Sinai and Lenox Hill Hospitals. A former president of the American Diabetes Association, New York Diabetes affiliate, he has been a member of the board of directors of the New York Diabetes Association. He was chosen Endocrinologist of the Year 2005 by the Division of Endocrinology, Diabetes and Bone Diseases at Mount Sinai School of Medicine.

Dr. Mirsky is also on the board of directors of the Joslin Diabetes Center, Inc., in Boston, and he is the chairman of the Nutrition Committee of Lenox Hill Hospital. A member of the Medical Advisory Board of the New York Chapter of the Juvenile Diabetes Foundation, he received the Humanitarian Award of the Juvenile Diabetes Foundation, New York Chapter, in 1994.

A Phi Beta Kappa graduate of the University of Michigan, he also graduated from Northwestern University Medical School and was a captain in the U.S. Air Force.

JOAN RATTNER HEILMAN is a respected journalist and author who has written more than a dozen books and hundreds of magazine and newspaper articles, many of them on health and medicine. A member of the American Society of Journalists and Authors and the Authors Guild, she is a graduate of Smith College and a former magazine editor. Collaborating with noted physicians, she has coauthored many books, including *Estrogen: The Facts Can Change Your Life; What Every Woman Should Know: Staying Healthy After 40; Having a Cesarean Baby; The Complete University Medical Diet; The Complete Book of Midwifery;* and *Growing Up Thin.*